Recent Advances in Enteral Nutrition

Special Issue Editors

Omorogieva Ojo
Joanne Brooke

MDPI • Basel • Beijing • Wuhan • Barcelona • Belgrade

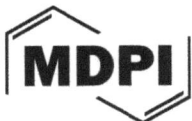

MDPI

Special Issue Editors
Omorogieva Ojo
University of Greenwich
UK

Joanne Brooke
University of Greenwich
UK

Editorial Office
MDPI AG
St. Alban-Anlage 66
Basel, Switzerland

This edition is a reprint of the Special Issue published online in the open access journal *Nutrients* (ISSN 2072-6643) in 2014–2016 (available at: http://www.mdpi.com/journal/nutrients/special_issues/advances-enteral-nutrition).

For citation purposes, cite each article independently as indicated on the article page online and as indicated below:

Lastname, F.M.; Lastname, F.M. Article title. *Journal Name*. **Year**. *Article number*, page range.

ISBN 978-3-03842-702-5 (Pbk)
ISBN 978-3-03842-701-8 (PDF)

Table of Contents

About the Special Issue Editors

Omorogieva Ojo has a PhD in nutrition from the university of Greenwich, London, a post graduate diploma in diabetes from university of Surrey, Roehampton and a graduate certificate in Higher Education from university of Greenwich. Prior to these qualifications, Dr Ojo had his BSc and MSc in animal science from university of Ibadan, Nigeria. He is currently a Senior Lecturer in Primary Care in the Faculty of Education and Health, university of Greenwich and he teaches across a range of courses and programmes. He was previously a nutrition specialist at the Home Enteral Nutrition Team, Lewisham Primary Care Trust, London, a post-doctoral research fellow in the School of Science, university of Greenwich, London and taught at College of Agriculture, Asaba, Nigeria. His key interest and areas of expertise are nutrition and diabetes which form the focus of his teaching and research activities including PhD supervision. Dr Ojos work is recognised both nationally and internationally and he has been a keynote speaker at international conferences and he is on the editorial board of six international journals including Nutrients.

Joanne Brooke is an Adult Nurse and a chartered Health Psychologist. Dr Brooke has a wealth of experience in healthcare, but has specialized in the care and support of older people and people with dementia. Dr Brooke is both an academic and clinician with recent posts as Nurse Consultant in Dementia for Kent Community NHS Foundation Trust and Associate Professor for University of West London and Royal Berkshire NHS Foundation Trust, and is currently a Reader in Older Persons Complex Care within the Oxford Institute of Nursing, Midwifery, and Allied Health Research, which is hosted by Oxford Brookes University. Dr Brooke is also the Director of the International Dementia and Culture Collaborative. Dr Brooke is on the editorial board of Journal of Clinical Nursing. As an academic Dr Brooke has been a speaker at international conferences specifically relating to dementia

Preface to "Recent Advances in Enteral Nutrition"

Welcome to the interesting topic of enteral nutrition. Healthcare professionals including nurses, doctors, nutritionists, dietitians and speech and language therapists who support people with nutritional deficit and/or swallowing difficulty recognize the need for enteral nutrition provision in order to meet the nutritional requirements of these patients. Therefore, this book provides an up-to-date research evidence covering the recent advances in enteral nutrition. It has been the result of the contribution of a number of experts in this field on a range of topical issues. These experts come from different parts of the world and specialize in different aspects of enteral nutrition which should provide the reader a better and broader understanding of this specialist area of nutrition.

The book is aimed at healthcare professionals and students involved in enteral nutrition support and research as well as patients who may require enteral tube feeding. The book has fourteen chapters. While the chapter on recent advances in enteral nutrition provides an overview of the broad perspectives of the various topics discussed in the book, the other chapters capture detailed narratives of original research and reviews that will guide healthcare professionals in their areas of practice. These include the use of enteral nutrition in a range of long term conditions such as diabetes, dementia and inflammatory bowel disease. In addition, discussion of the challenges of home enteral tube feeding and the developments and evaluation of the home enteral nutrition team which are essential for community enteral nutrition provision are some of the key elements of the book.

Omorogieva Ojo, Joanne Brooke
Special Issue Editors

nutrients

MDPI

Review

Recent Advances in Enteral Nutrition

Omorogieva Ojo [1],* and Joanne Brooke [2]

[1] Senior Lecturer in Primary Care, Faculty of Education and Health, University of Greenwich, London SE9 2UG, UK

[2] Reader in Complex Older Persons care Oxford Institute of Nursing and Allied Health Research, Faculty of health and Life Sciences, Oxford Brookes University, Oxford OX3 0FL, UK; jbrooke@brookes.ac.uk

* Correspondence: o.ojo@greenwich.ac.uk; Tel.: +44-20-8331-8626; Fax: +44-20-8331-8060

Received: 31 October 2016; Accepted: 2 November 2016; Published: 8 November 2016

There have been significant advances in the provision of enteral nutrition support in the acute and community healthcare settings. Enteral nutrition is beneficial to individuals who have functional guts but may not be able to meet their nutritional requirements via a normal diet. Most of these people have neurological conditions such as stroke, multiple sclerosis and dementia which could impact on swallowing reflexes, leading to dysphagia [1]. Others may have cancer, intellectual disability or conditions such as HIV and failure to thrive.

Therefore, the provision of nutrition support in the form of oral nutritional supplements (ONS) and enteral nutrition support can help mitigate the challenges of nutritional deficit [2]. Enteral feeding can be delivered via a range of feeding tubes and through different methods of feeding including continuous, bolus and gravity feeding [3]. While nasogastric tube (NGT) feeding is often provided to individuals requiring short-term enteral nutrition provision, the percutaneous endoscopic gastrostomy (PEG) tube is for long-term enteral feeding [4]. For individuals with partial/complete gastrectomy and those who are at higher risk of aspiration, the use of the jejunostomy feeding tube may help alleviate these problems [5]. On the other hand, the radiologically inserted gastrostomy (RIG) tube may be the tube of choice in head and neck cancer patients who may have high risk of malignant cell translocation from the primary site of disease to the stoma site. Similarly, the use of the balloon gastrostomy feeding tube, following the dislodgement of the conventional enteral feeding tube (PEG, RIG), is common, although there is evidence that the balloon gastrostomy feeding tube is now used as a primary tube of choice in head and neck cancer patients [6].

Usually, the provision of enteral nutrition entails nutritional status assessment and the evaluation of nutritional requirements of patients [7]. In addition, the development of feeding regimes, protocols, guidelines, algorithms, and the management of patients, pumps, feeds, and feeding tubes are essential aspects of enteral nutrition provision.

The developments in enteral nutrition appear to center on many aspects, including the increasing use of enteral feeding in patients with long-term conditions, the development of multidisciplinary teams including extended roles for dietitians and nurses and the use of guidelines. This may not be unrelated to the worldwide increase in the aging population and increasing prevalence of long-term conditions with associated complications, resulting in swallowing difficulties and malnutrition [8].

Therefore, the essence of the Special Issue on Recent Advances in Enteral Nutrition was to capture key developments in this area of research and practice. For instance, dementia is a long-term condition that impacts on people's cognitive and physical abilities which can affect their nutritional intake, leading to malnutrition [9]. Malnutrition in patients with dementia appears to correlate with cognitive decline and the progression of the disease. The use of percutaneous endoscopic gastrostomy which is used widely in supporting patients with a range of conditions seems to be discouraged in dementia care [10]. In a systematic review on the use of enteral nutrition in patients with advanced dementia, Finucane et al. [10] did not find any improvements in the rates of aspiration, pressure sores and mortality and therefore concluded that enteral nutrition for patients with dementia should be discouraged [10]. In contrast, recent recommendations from the systematic review by Brooke and Ojo [9] challenged this position and instead suggested the need for a holistic assessment of patients with dementia requiring enteral nutrition and PEG tube placement. These assessments should include a diagnosis of patients—comorbidities, current stage of dementia, acute medical illness and its impact on nutritional status [9].

Another area where enteral nutrition is being used to support patients with a long-term condition is in diabetes care and management. The complications of diabetes are wide ranging and may include stroke, which could impact on the swallowing ability of the individuals [4]. The use of enteral nutrition to support these people who are unable to meet their nutritional requirements via oral intake alone becomes imperative [11]. Therefore, Ojo and Brooke [12] evaluated the use of standard and diabetes specific enteral formulas in the management of diabetes in a systematic review. Based on the response of blood glucose and other parameters including HBA1c in the studies reviewed, it was concluded that the use of diabetes specific formula may be effective in managing glucose in patients with diabetes and on enteral nutrition [12].

There have been advances in the use of enteral nutrition to support patients with head and neck cancer and other cancers through the use of different feeding tubes, both as prophylactic and reactive treatments [13,14]. Patients with head and neck cancer are mostly malnourished and/or at risk of malnutrition, therefore, prophylactic feeding through NGT or PEG aimed at improving weight gain and promoting hydration is now common [15]. However, based on the narrative review by Bossola [15], it would appear that the use of prophylactic enteral feeding does not offer advantages with respect to nutritional outcomes, effect on radiotherapy treatment and survival compared with reactive feeding, which involves patients being offered NGT or PEG when oral nutritional supplements are inadequate in maintaining nutritional status [15].

In another study, Wang et al. [16] compared postoperative enteral nutrition with delayed enteral nutrition in patients with oesophageal cancer with a view to establishing the most appropriate time to commence enteral nutrition provision. It was concluded that early enteral nutrition started within 48 hours was safe for postoperative oesophageal cancer patients [16]. Based on this study, it was shown that early enteral nutrition is effective in reducing the incidence of postoperative pulmonary infection, promoting postoperative nutrition status, enhancing early recovery of intestinal movement and reducing the length of hospital stay and hospital cost [16].

Apart from patients with head and neck cancer, enteral nutrition is also used to support patients with other forms of cancer including pancreatic cancer. According to Buscemi et al. [17], pancreaticoduodenectomy is used for the treatment of periampullory carcinomas and patients who have undertaken this procedure are often malnourished with significant impact on postoperative wound healing and recovery. Following this review, it was concluded that enteral nutrition appeared safe and tolerated by patients who have had pancreaticoduodenectomy although it did not provide any advantage in terms of postoperative pancreatic fistula, postpancreatectomy haemorrhage, length of hospital stay and infectious complications [17].

Inflammatory bowel disease, which includes at least three clinical conditions (ulcerative colitis, Crohn's disease and indeterminate colitis), is another condition that may benefit from advances in enteral nutrition support [18]. There is evidence that malnutrition is a common effect of inflammatory bowel disease and diet has been implicated in its pathogenesis and clinical manifestation [18]. In addition, diet also has a role in the management of inflammatory bowel disease and the need for enteral nutrition support becomes critical when oral dietary intake is not sufficient to offer all the nutritional requirements [19]. Enteral nutrition has shown promising results in the management of Crohn's disease as it provides equal or higher remission rates than current medications in use [18].

In a related study, exclusive enteral nutrition—the monotonous enteral delivery of complete liquid nutrition—has been explored in the management of Crohn's disease [19]. Exclusive enteral nutrition is usually in the form of liquid enteral formulas which may be elemental (e.g., in the form of amino acids) or polymeric (e.g., in the form of intact protein) [19]. Although the mechanism of action of exclusive enteral nutrition is still evolving, there is evidence that it could modify the composition of intestinal microbiome which are essential in the pathogenesis of Crohn's disease [19]. It would appear that exclusive enteral nutrition is better than steroids in the induction of mucosal healing and may provide long-term remission in some cases of Crohn's disease [19].

The efficacy and safety of the use of an enteral immunomodulatory diet (omega-3 fatty acid, γ-linolenic acid and antioxidant supplementation) for acute lung injury and acute respiratory distress syndrome are also areas of interest in enteral nutrition provision. This view relies on the understanding that this therapy may be used for the treatment of these conditions, although researchers are not unanimous on this position [20]. Based on the current systematic review [20], it is now clear that an enteral immunomodulatory diet could not reduce the severity of acute lung injury and acute respiratory distress syndrome.

In Very Low Birth Weight (VLBW) infants, feeding methods in enteral nutrition have been explored based on the observation that continuous enteral feeding methodmay result in significant loss of fat and micronutrients [21]. Therefore, Tabata et al. [21] examined the fat loss in enteral nutrition based on the current methods of providing fortified human milk in high risk infants. In addition, the study evaluated whether fortifier and cream improved fat delivery in continuous enteral infant feeding of breast milk [21]. Based on this study, it was clear that fat and nutrient loss in continuous enteral feeding was presenting a challenge to the provision of nutrients to Very Low Birth Weight infants [21]. Therefore, the bolus feeding method is recommended where possible and for infants who are unable to tolerate bolus feeding, the addition of fortifiers and/or cream to human milk, in order to increase fat percentage, is recommended [21].

The use of human milk fortified with donor human milk-derived fortifier (HMDF) in premature infants has been reported to increase serum phosphorus although the evidence appears anedoctal [22]. Therefore, the study by Chetta et al. [22] investigated this phenomenon and concluded that the incidence of elevated serum phosphorus was mild and not permanent in premature infants receiving human milk with HMDF.

Despite the merits of enteral nutrition, there are a number of challenges militating against the use of enteral feeding. These include problems of funding, inadequate or lack of standards, policies, management approaches, guidelines and infrastructure for the delivery of enteral nutrition [23]. Therefore, strategies for ameliorating these challenges should include the development of the Home Enteral Nutrition (HEN) service which should promote multi-disciplinary team working and the development of national and international standards and guidelines [23]. The National Institute for Health and Care Excellence (NICE) guidance on nutrition support [24] emphasizes the quality standard for nutrition support in adults and stresses the need for all care services to be responsible in identifying those who are at risk of malnutrition and providing nutrition support for the people who need it. In addition, Dutta et al. [25] conducted a comprehensive literature review and developed a set of guidelines for feeding Very Low Birth Weight (VLBW) infants. It was concluded that there is a need to aim for full feeds at about 2 weeks of age in neonates weighing <1000 g at birth and for 1 week in those neonates weighing 1000–1500 g at birth [25]. The use of trophic feeds (10–15 mL/kg/day) should commence within 24 h of birth although caution is required in extremely pre-term, extremely low birth weight and infants with growth restriction [25].

The development of multidisciplinary teams, including primary care teams involved in enteral nutrition provisions, has been shown to improve cost effectiveness [26]. A Home Enteral Nutrition team comprising dietitians, nurses and speech and language therapist has the potential to improve patient satisfaction and reduce the costs which are associated with enteral tube feeding in the community [27]. This is often achieved through the development and implementation of care pathways for the management of patients on enteral tube feeding by the HEN team and effective multidisciplinary team working [26]. The use of the HEN service has increased significantly in the past few decades and this has led to the development of various policies and guidelines for the management of enteral nutrition [28]. This has also contributed to the promotion of multidisciplinary team working and the extension of roles of the different professionals that make up the HEN team [27,29].

Conflicts of Interest: The authors declare no conflict of interest.

References

1. Rowat, A. Enteral tube feeding for dysphagic stroke patients. *Br. J. Nurs.* **2015**, *24*, 138–144. [CrossRef]
2. Ojo, O. The use of oral nutritional supplements in the acute care setting. *Br. J. Nurs.* **2016**, *25*, 664–666. [CrossRef]
3. Parker, E.K.; Faruquie, S.S.; Talbot, P. Trends in home enteral nutrition at a tertiary teaching hospital: 2005–2013. *Nutr. Diet.* **2015**, *72*, 267–275. [CrossRef]
4. Catangui, E.J.; Slark, J. Nurse led ward rounds: A valuable contribution to acute stroke care. *Br. J. Nurs.* **2012**, *21*, 801–805. [CrossRef]
5. Ojo, O. Problems with use of a Foley catheter in home enteral tube feeding. *Br. J. Nurs.* **2014**, *23*, 360–364. [CrossRef]
6. Ojo, O. Balloon gastrostomy tubes for long-term feeding in the community. *Br. J. Nurs.* **2011**, *20*, 34–38. [CrossRef]
7. National Institute for Health and Care Excellence (NICE). Nutrition Support for Adults: Oral Nutrition Support, Enteral Tube Feeding and Parenteral Nutrition (CG32). 2006. Available online: https://www.nice.org.uk/guidance/cg32 (accessed on 1 October 2016).
8. Ferri, C.P.; Prince, M.; Brayne, C.; Brodaty, H.; Fratiglioni, L.; Ganguli, M.; Hall, K.; Hasegawa, K.; Hendrie, H.; Huang, Y.; et al. Global prevalence of dementia: A Delphi consensus study. *Lancet* **2005**, *366*, 2112–2117. [CrossRef]
9. Brooke, J.; Ojo, O. Enteral Nutrition in Dementia: A Systematic Review. *Nutrients* **2015**, *7*, 2456–2468. [CrossRef]
10. Finucance, T.E.; Christmas, C.; Travis, K. Tube feeding in patients with advanced dementia: A review of the evidence. *JAMA* **1999**, *282*, 1365–1370. [CrossRef]
11. Mahoney, C.; Rowat, A.; Macmillan, M.; Dennis, M. Nasogastric feeding for stroke patients: Practice and education. *Br. J. Nurs.* **2015**, *24*, 319–320. [CrossRef]
12. Ojo, O.; Brooke, J. Evaluation of the Role of Enteral Nutrition in Managing Patients with Diabetes: A Systematic Review. *Nutrients* **2014**, *6*, 5142–5152. [CrossRef]
13. Sheth, C.H.; Sharp, S.; Walters, E.R. Enteral feeding in head and neck cancer patients at a UK cancer centre. *J. Hum. Nutr. Diet.* **2013**, *26*, 421–428. [CrossRef]
14. Nugent, B.; Parker, M.; McIntyre, I. Nasogastric tube feeding and percutaneous endoscopic gastrostomy tube feeding in patients with head and neck cancer. *J. Hum. Nutr. Diet.* **2010**, *23*, 277–284. [CrossRef]
15. Bossola, M. Nutritional Interventions in Head and Neck Cancer Patients Undergoing Chemoradiotherapy: A Narrative Review. *Nutrients* **2015**, *7*, 265–276. [CrossRef]
16. Wang, G.; Chen, H.; Liu, J.; Ma, Y.; Jia, H. A Comparison of Postoperative Early Enteral Nutrition with Delayed Enteral Nutrition in Patients with Esophageal Cancer. *Nutrients* **2015**, *7*, 4308–4317. [CrossRef]
17. Buscemi, S.; Damiano, G.; Palumbo, V.D.; Spinelli, G.; Ficarella, S.; Monte, G.L.; Marrazzo, A.; Monte, A.I.L. Enteral Nutrition in Pancreaticoduodenectomy: A Literature Review. *Nutrients* **2015**, *7*, 3154–3165. [CrossRef]
18. Altomare, R.; Damiano, G.; Abruzzo, A.; Palumbo, V.D.; Tomasello, G.; Buscemi, S.; Lo Monte, A.I. Enteral Nutrition Support to Treat Malnutrition in Inflammatory Bowel Disease. *Nutrients* **2015**, *7*, 2125–2133. [CrossRef]
19. Shah, R.; Kellermayer, R. Microbiome Associations of Therapeutic Enteral Nutrition. *Nutrients* **2014**, *6*, 5298–5311. [CrossRef]
20. Li, C.; Bo, L.; Liu, W.; Lu, X.; Jin, F. Enteral Immunomodulatory Diet (Omega-3 Fatty Acid, γ-Linolenic Acid and Antioxidant Supplementation) for Acute Lung Injury and Acute Respiratory Distress Syndrome: An Updated Systematic Review and Meta-Analysis. *Nutrients* **2015**, *7*, 5572–5585. [CrossRef]
21. Tabata, M.; Abdelrahman, K.; Hair, A.B.; Hawthorne, K.M.; Chen, Z.; Abrams, S.A. Fortifier and Cream Improve Fat Delivery in Continuous Enteral Infant Feeding of Breast Milk. *Nutrients* **2015**, *7*, 1174–1183. [CrossRef]

22. Chetta, K.E.; Hair, A.B.; Hawthorne, K.M.; Abrams, S.A. Serum Phosphorus Levels in Premature Infants Receiving a Donor Human Milk Derived Fortifier. *Nutrients* **2015**, *7*, 2562–2573. [CrossRef]

23. Ojo, O. The Challenges of Home Enteral Tube Feeding: A Global Perspective. *Nutrients* **2015**, *7*, 2524–2538. [CrossRef]

24. National Institute for Health and Care Excellence (NICE). *Nutrition Support in Adults Quality*; Standard [QS24]; NICE: London, UK, 2012.

25. Dutta, S.; Singh, B.; Chessell, L.; Wilson, J.; Janes, M.; McDonald, K.; Shahid, S.; Gardner, V.A. Hjartarson, A.; Purcha, M.; et al. Guidelines for Feeding Very Low Birth Weight Infants. *Nutrients* **2015**, *7*, 423–442. [CrossRef]

26. Dinenage, S.; Gower, M.; van Wyk, J.; Blamey, A.; Ashbolt, K.; Sutcliffe, M.; Green, S.M. Development and Evaluation of a Home Enteral Nutrition Team. *Nutrients* **2015**, *7*, 1607–1617. [CrossRef]

27. Ojo, O.; Patel, I. Home enteral nutrition and team working. *J. Community Nurs.* **2012**, *26*, 15–18.

28. De Luis, D.A.; Izaola, O.; Cuellar, L.A.; Terroba, M.C.; Cabezas, G.; De La Fuente, B. Experience over 12 years with home enteral nutrition in a healthcare area of Spain. *J. Hum. Nutr. Diet.* **2013**, *26* (Suppl. 1), 39–44. [CrossRef]

29. Stanley, W.; Borthwick, A.M. Extended roles and the dietitian: Community adult enteral tube care. *J. Hum. Nutr. Diet.* **2013**, *26*, 298–305. [CrossRef]

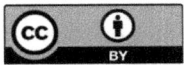

nutrients

MDPI

Review

Evaluation of the Role of Enteral Nutrition in Managing Patients with Diabetes: A Systematic Review

Omorogieva Ojo * and Joanne Brooke

Faculty of Education and Health, University of Greenwich, Avery Hill Road, Avery Hill Campus, London, SE9 2UG, UK; J.M.Brooke@greenwich.ac.uk

* Author to whom correspondence should be addressed; o.ojo@greenwich.ac.uk; Tel.: +44-(0)20-8331-8626; Fax: +44-(0)20-8331-8060.

Received: 29 September 2014; in revised form: 14 October 2014; Accepted: 17 October 2014; Published: 18 November 2014

Abstract: The aim of this systematic review is to evaluate the role of enteral nutrition in managing patients with diabetes on enteral feed. The prevalence of diabetes is on the increase in the UK and globally partly due to lack of physical activities, poor dietary regimes and genetic susceptibility. The development of diabetes often leads to complications such as stroke, which may require enteral nutritional support. The provision of enteral feeds comes with its complications including hyperglycaemia which if not managed can have profound consequences for the patients in terms of clinical outcomes. Therefore, it is essential to develop strategies for managing patients with diabetes on enteral feed with respect to the type and composition of the feed. This is a systematic review of published peer reviewed articles. EBSCOhost Research, PubMed and SwetsWise databases were searched. Reference lists of identified articles were reviewed. Randomised controlled trials comparing enteral nutrition diabetes specific formulas with standard formulas were included. The studies which compared diabetes specific formulas (DSF) with standard formulas showed that DSF was more effective in controlling glucose profiles including postprandial glucose, HbA1c and insulinemic response. The use of DSF appears to be effective in managing patients with diabetes on enteral feed compared with standard feed.

Keywords: enteral nutrition; diabetes; diabetes specific formula; standard formula; hyperglycaemia; glycaemic index

1. Introduction

The prevalence of diabetes and the cost to the National Health Service (NHS) have been on the increase in the UK [1,2]. Various factors including the failure to maintain a healthy lifestyle such as regular physical activity and healthy dietary regimes, and genetic susceptibility have been ascribed as possible reasons for the high incidence of the condition [3,4]. The manifestation of diabetes comes with various complications such as cerebrovascular accident, which may result in dysphagia, often requiring nutritional support [5,6]. This is especially evident in patients with diabetes who may be unable to maintain their nutritional requirements through the use of oral dietary intake alone and thus may require enteral feed. In addition, their involvement in physical activity that would ensure the maintenance of normal glucose levels may be compromised due to their neurological conditions and poor mobility [7,8]. Therefore, managing a person with diabetes on enteral nutrition could present some difficulties for the multidisciplinary healthcare professional (HCP) team if there are no effective strategies for managing the enteral feed [9]. There could be increased risk of the patient with diabetes on enteral feed developing hyperglycaemia or hypoglycaemia, which can result in potentially poorer clinical outcomes [10–12].

In a study by Ojo [13], comparison of patients on home enteral tube feeding (HETF) with the Quality and Outcome Framework (QOF) data revealed that diabetes prevalence in people on HEFT in Lambeth, Lewisham and Southwark primary care trusts in the UK was significantly higher (7.78%) than in the general population (3.63%) not on enteral nutrition and living in the same area. Ojo [13] showed that more patients who have diabetes are now requiring enteral nutrition support.

The role of enteral nutrition in patients with diabetes is to provide the required macro- and micro-nutrients including energy, protein, vitamins and minerals in part or whole in order to reduce the risk of malnutrition in these patients [14]. However, due to the nature of the different food formulas, the risk of hyperglycemia could be a major challenge in these patients and newly diagnosed hyperglycaemia could be considered an independent prognostic factor of mortality in patients with enteral feeding [15,16]. Hyperglycaemia can have profound impacts on a range of patients with diabetes including those hospitalised, such as patients with diabetic ulcers or undergoing limb amputations. Hyperglycemia may impact on wound healing, time spent in hospital and lead to complications including diabetic ketoacidosis and hyperosmolar non-ketotic state [17,18]. Therefore, there is the need to ensure adequate management of patients with diabetes, especially those on enteral feed because of the effects on blood glucose levels. The cost of major complications resulting from hyperglycaemia to the UK economy has been estimated to be between £872 for blindness in one eye to £8459 for amputation per patient, although the total cost of type 2 diabetes to the UK economy appears difficult to evaluate [19]. However, in 2007 estimates of 7%–12% of the total NHS budget, which could be £2.8 billion associated cost for the UK has been reported [1,20].

Nutritional requirements of patients with diabetes on enteral nutrition are met with the use of standard enteral feeds or diabetes specific feeds. Diabetes specific formulas contain specific ingredients that often include fructose and a large amount of monounsaturated fatty acids, which are aimed at controlling postprandial glucose [21,22]. The effects of these feeds in maintaining the nutritional requirements and physiological state of patients with diabetes continue to generate debate and attract the interest of researchers. A scoping exercise of the literature revealed two systematic reviews on the role of enteral nutritional support and the use of diabetes specific formulas for patients with diabetes carried out at various times with different findings [19]. A systematic review and meta-analysis of enteral nutritional support and use of diabetes specific formulas conducted by Elia *et al.* [19] aimed to determine the benefits of nutritional support in patients with types 1 and 2 diabetes. It compared the use of nutritional support with routine care, and standard formulas with diabetes formulas. Although the study concluded that the use of diabetes specific formulas (DSF) as oral nutrition supplements and tube feeds improve blood glucose levels when compared with standard formulas, controversies still surround the use of DSF. In particular, there are clinical interests in establishing the safety and tolerance of relatively high levels of fat and fructose in patients with underlying dysmotility disorders such as irritable bowel syndrome and with respect to lipid metabolism and lactic acidosis [22]. Since the study by Elia *et al.* [19], a number of randomised controlled trials based on patients with diabetes on enteral nutrition have been published. In addition, the American Society of Parenteral and Enteral Nutrition (ASPEN) Clinical Guidelines: nutrition support of adult patients with hyperglycaemia which was developed in order to provide the desired blood glucose goal in hospitalized patients receiving nutritional support could not recommend whether diabetes specific formulas can be used for hospitalised adult patients with hyperglycaemia [23].

The ASPEN Clinical Guidelines recommendation for the use of diabetes specific formula was based on only two studies published in 2003 and 2005. It was therefore not surprising that the ASPEN guideline recommended that further research was required in the use of diabetic specific formulas [23]. According to Cheng [24], two strategies for managing hyperglycaemia of enteral feeding are adjustment of the enteral feed carbohydrate content and pharmacological therapy to lower glucose levels although the current review is focused on the former.

Drawing from the above reviews and guidelines, the need to examine the role of standard *versus* diabetes specific formulas has become pertinent. Therefore, the aim of the present study is to carry out a systematic review of the role of enteral nutrition in supporting patients with diabetes. However, the use of insulin and oral hypoglycaemic agents was not examined in this review.

The objective is as follows:

- To examine the effects of standard and diabetes specific enteral formulas in the management of diabetes.

The research question is:

- Is diabetes specific formula more effective than standard formulas in managing patients with diabetes on enteral feed?

2. Experimental Section

A systematic review was carried out based on published guidelines [25,26]. This involved a literature search of articles of interest relating to the use of enteral nutrition in diabetes management, including a general scoping of the data bases which found only two systematic reviews that were relevant to the population and intervention of interest. A search of the Cochraine library and databases of abstracts of reviews and effects found one article by Elia *et al.* [19], which was published in 2005. A further search of SwetsWise and EBSCO host databases found the ASPEN guidelines; nutrition support of adult patients with hyperglycaemia [23]. Although this guideline was published in 2013, it derived most of its limited evidence with respect to the question on the use of diabetes specific formulas in adult hospitalised patients with hyperglycaemia from studies published between 2003 and 2005.

The research question was defined into the component parts; the Population (P), the Interventions (I), Comparative interventions (C) and Outcomes (O) based on PICO framework [25]. Table 1 shows the results of the various searches. The databases searched included EBSCO Host/Health Sciences Research databases (encompassing Academic search premier, Medline, Psychology and Behavioural sciences collection, PSYCINFO, SPORTDISCUSS and Cumulative Index to Nursing and Allied Health Literature (CINAHL) Plus) and SwetsWise. The reference list of relevant systematic reviews and articles were checked in order to identify studies that could be useful to the present review.

Table 1. Literature search strategy.

Database	Dates Covered	Date Searched	Hits	Search Terms
EBSCO Host (Health Sciences Research Databases)	2005–2014	04.06.14	469,184	Diabetes
EBSCO Host (Health Sciences Research Databases)	2005–2014	04.06.14	323	Diabetes and Enteral Nutrition
EBSCO Host (Health Sciences Research Databases)	2005–2014	04.06.14	13	Diabetes and Enteral Nutrition and Diabetes Specific formula
EBSCO Host (Health Sciences Research Databases)	2005–2014	04.06.14	2	Diabetes and Enteral Nutrition and Standard Feed
EBSCO Host (Health Sciences Research Databases)	2005–2014	04.06.14	1	Diabetes and Enteral Nutrition and Glycated Haemoglobin
EBSCO Host (Health Sciences Research Databases)	2005–2014	04.06.14	4	Diabetes and Enteral Nutrition and Fasting Blood Glucose
EBSCO Host (Health Sciences Research Databases)	2005–2014	04.06.14	28	Diabetes and Enteral Nutrition and Hyperglycaemia
EBSCO Host (Health Sciences Research Databases)	2005–2014	04.06.14	11	Diabetes and Enteral Nutrition and Hypoglycaemia
SwetsWise	2005–2014	04.06.14	46	Diabetes and Enteral Nutrition
SwetsWise	2005–2014	04.06.14	47	Diabetes and Standard feed
SwetsWise	2005–2014	04.06.14	73	Diabetes and Diabetes Specific feed

2.1. Inclusion and Exclusion Criteria

Only randomised controlled trials were selected for inclusion in the current review.

The participants in the studies included in the systematic review were adult males and females who had diabetes and were on enteral nutrition while the interventions were standard enteral feed and DSF.

The outcome measures included in the search were; HbA1c, fasting blood glucose, hyperglycaemia and hypoglycaemia.

In terms of the years of publication, searches were conducted between 2005 and 2014 while only studies written in English language were included. Studies that did not meet the above inclusion criteria were excluded from the study.

2.2. Data Analysis

Based on the criteria outlined for exclusion and inclusion of various studies, 469,184 articles were initially available. This number was further reduced to 323 articles with the inclusion of enteral nutrition as part of the search term (Table 1). Of these articles, five articles that met the requirements for selection were included in the review (Table 2).

3. Results

All the studies included in the systematic review involved patients who had type 2 diabetes and these were clearly specified in the method section in the respective studies. While three studies compared DSF with standard formula [21,27,28], one study [29] compared slowly digested carbohydrate formula with DSF and standard formula (Table 2). The final study compared diabetes specific enteral formula with 49.95% calories provided by fat and diabetes specific enteral formula with 34% calories provided by fat [30].

In the study by Ceriello *et al.* [21], glucose profiles were significantly better after administering DSF compared with standard formula. In addition, diabetes specific formula significantly improved postprandial glucose compared with the standard, fibre-containing formula.

With respect to the study by Vaisman *et al.* [28], HbA1c decreased over time in the diabetes specific diet group and increased in the standard feed group. Similarly, in the randomised double-blinded study evaluating the postprandial glycaemic and insulinemic response conducted by Alish *et al.* [27], differences in adjusted peak plasma glucose levels were significantly lower in DSF compared with standard formulas (STF) ($p < 0.001$). In addition, differences in adjusted peak insulin levels were significantly lower in DSF compared with STF ($p = 0.017$). In other words, the use of DSF produced significantly lower postprandial and insulinemic response.

Voss [29] revealed that adjusted glucose concentrations were significantly higher at all points after feeding the STF compared with the slowly digested carbohydrate formula (SDC) or DSF ($p < 0.001$). In addition, adjusted plasma glucose concentrations for the SDC were observed to be significantly lower than those for the DSF from 30 to 120 min ($p < 0.05$). In relation to the adjusted insulin responses, these were significantly higher for the STF compared with the SDC at each time point, while the SDC had a significantly lower insulinemic response compared with the DSF at 90 and 120 min ($p < 0.05$) [29]. Finally, the adjusted results for postprandial glucagon-like polypeptide-1 (GLP-1) levels at 30 and 60 min in this study were significantly lower for the STF compared with SDC ($p < 0.05$), but not different from the DSF [29].

In the study by De Luis *et al.* [30] which compared diabetes specific enteral supplement with 49.95% calories provided by fat (Gp 1) and diabetes specific enteral supplement with 34% calories provided by fat (Gp 2), a significant decrease of glucose and HbA1c was observed in Gp 1 compared with Gp 2.

Table 2. Summary of studies reviewed.

Citation	Study Type	Population and Sample Size	Age (Years)	Intervention	Outcomes	Remarks
Ceriello A et al., 2009 [21]	Randomized Controlled Study	12	67.2 ± 1.3	Diabetes-Specific Formula (DSF) / Standard Formula (STF)	Fasting Glucose (mmol/L) = 7.9 ± 0.45; 24 h Glucose Concentrate (mmol/L-SEM) = 8.7 ± 0.5; Day time = 9.4 ± 0.6; Fasting Glucose (mmol/L) = 7.6 ± 0.37; 24 h Glucose Conc. (mmol/L-SEM) = 9.6 ± 0.6; Day time = 10.7 ± 0.6	Results are expressed as mean ± SEM
Voss AC, 2008 [29]	Randomized Controlled Study	48	56 ± 1.4 (SEM)	Slowly Digested Carbohydrate Formula (SDC) / DSF STF	The positive area under the curve for glucose and insulin with STF was higher ($p < 0.001$) compared with the SDC and DSF. The adjusted Glucagon-like peptide-1 (GLP-1) concentration at 60 min. was higher for the SDC compared with the DSF and STF ($p < 0.05$).	Results are expressed as mean ± SEM
De Luis et al., 2008 [30]	Randomized Clinical Trial	16 / 14	74.6 ± 7.1 / 77.1 ± 8.7	Diabetes Specific Enteral Formula (49.95% of Calories provided by fat, Gp 1) / Diabetes Specific Enteral Formula (34% of Calories provided by fat, Gp 2)	Baseline Glucose mg/dL = 119.8 ± 42 10 weeks = 95.1 ± 16.8 HbA1c% = 8.2 ± 2.8 at baseline, 5.8 ± 0.7% at 10 weeks; Baseline Glucose mg/dL = 122.4 ± 22.8 10 weeks = 130.6 ± 41.4; Baseline HbA1c% = 7.58 ± 1.7 10 weeks = 7.38 ± 1.5	Results are expressed as mean ± SD
Vaisman et al., 2009 [28]	Randomized Controlled Trial	13 / 12	79.2 ± 10.4 (Mean ± SD) / 73.0 ± 14.7 (Mean ± SD)	Standard tube feed / Diabetes Specific Tube feed	HbA1c = 7.9 ± 0.3% at baseline, 8.7 ± 0.4% at 12 weeks; HbA1c = 6.9 ± 0.3% at baseline, 6.2 ± 0.4% at 12 weeks	Results are expressed as mean ± SEM
Alish CJ et al., 2010 [27]	Randomized, double blinded crossover design (Postprandial glycaemic and Insulinemic response)	22	63.1 ± 1.9	DSFs / STFs	Baseline plasma Glucose = 113.1 ± 6.9 mg/dL. Adjusted (change from baseline) plasma glucose conc. = 22.3 ± 4.4 mg/dL. Baseline insulin levels = 21.2 ± 2.9 μL/mL. Peak insulin levels = 79.5 ± 17.2 μL/mL. Baseline plasma Glucose = 124.8 ± 5.3 mg/dL. Adjusted (change from baseline) plasma glucose conc. = 71.1 ± 7.0 mg/dL. Baseline insulin levels = 16.3 ± 1.7 μL/mL. Peak insulin levels = 115.2 ± 28.0 μL/mL.	Results are expressed as mean ± SEM

With respect to the study by Vaisman *et al.* [28], HbA1c decreased over time in the diabetes specific diet group and increased in the standard feed group. Similarly, in the randomised double-blinded study evaluating the postprandial glycaemic and insulinemic response conducted by Alish *et al.* [27], differences in adjusted peak plasma glucose levels were significantly lower in DSF compared with STF ($p < 0.001$). In addition, differences in adjusted peak insulin levels were significantly lower in DSF compared with STF ($p = 0.017$). In other words, the use of DSF produced significantly lower postprandial and insulinemic response.

Voss [29] revealed that adjusted glucose concentrations were significantly higher at all points after feeding the STF compared with the SDC or DSF ($p < 0.001$). In addition, adjusted plasma glucose concentrations for the SDC were observed to be significantly lower than those for the DSF from 30 to 120 min ($p < 0.05$). In relation to the adjusted insulin responses, these were significantly higher for the STF compared with the SDC at each time point, while the SDC had a significantly lower insulinemic response compared with the DSF at 90 and 120 min ($p < 0.05$) [29]. Finally, the adjusted results for postprandial GLP-1 levels at 30 and 60 min in this study were significantly lower for the STF compared with SDC ($p < 0.05$), but not different from the DSF [29].

In the study by De Luis *et al.* [30] which compared diabetes specific enteral supplement with 49.95% calories provided by fat (Gp 1) and diabetes specific enteral supplement with 34% calories provided by fat (Gp 2), a significant decrease of glucose and HbA1c was observed in Gp 1 compared with Gp 2.

4. Discussion

Diabetes specific formula seems to be effective in managing glucose profiles including postprandial glucose and insulinemic response and HbA1c compared with standard formula in patients with diabetes on enteral nutrition. The effectiveness of DSF in patients with diabetes on enteral feed may be partly due to the form of carbohydrate used in its formulation. Diabetes specific formulas often contain carbohydrate that are more slowly digested and absorbed compared with standard formula that contain carbohydrates that are more rapidly digested and absorbed [27]. Postprandial blood glucose response, which is a risk factor for micro- and macro-vascular complications, has been shown to be influenced profoundly by the specific composition of the diet [31]. The measure of how soon glucose reaches the blood stream is often termed the glycaemic index (GI) of food while the glycaemic load (GL) shows the overall glycaemic effect of a specific amount of food item [1]. It is possible that DSFs are formulated with carbohydrates which have lower GI compared with standard formulas. In a study conducted by Hofman *et al.* [32], it was shown that the GI of the 12 enteral formulas determined in the study varied widely from GI = 12 for a diabetes specific feed up to GI = 61 for a standard supplement. High GI foods have GI value ≥70 while medium GI values range from 55 to 70 compared to low GI foods that have GI value ≤55 [33]. According to Hofman *et al.* [32], in general, a low GI formula (DSF) is characterised by reduced carbohydrate content, presence of fructose, a higher fat content containing monounsaturated fatty acids (MUFA) and high amounts of fibre while standard formulas, especially sip feeds, often do not contain fibre. This view is reinforced by Charney and Hertzler [34] who noted that diets containing up to 30% of total calories as MUFA have led to improvements in lipoprotein levels and glycaemic control in patients with diabetes. In addition, small doses of fructose (5 g to 10 g) have been found to be effective in reducing acute glycaemic response to a carbohydrate challenge partly because of the low GI of fructose, which is 19 compared with the GI of glucose which is 100 [34]. On the other hand, standard enteral formulas, whether oral or enteral, are high in carbohydrate, low in fat and fibres compared with DSFs which contain defined nutrient composition such as fructose, fibre, MUFA, soy bean and antioxidants which are designed to improve glycaemic control [19]. The source of carbohydrate in DSF includes increased amount of fructose relative to standard formulas and fat often in the form of higher amounts MUFA when compared with standard formulas although issues around tolerance on high levels of fats and fructose in feed have been subjects of discussion [22,35]. The main sources of fibre in DSF are usually fruits and vegetables and the levels are relatively higher than in standard formulas.

Nutrients **2014**, *6*, 5142–5152

Evidence of a meta-analaysis demonstrates that low GI foods have clinically more useful effect on medium-term glycaemic control (glycated proteins) in patients with diabetes [32]. According to Widanagamage *et al.* [36], the long-term use of foods that have high GI can place a higher metabolic demand on the body in terms of higher insulin requirement with the potential to lead to insulin resistance.

5. Conclusions

The outcomes of the studies that compared Diabetes specific formula with standard formulas appear to show a trend with respect to the response of glucose and other parameters such as HbA1c, which define diabetes. Based on the evidence in the present review, there are indications that the use of Diabetes specific formula could be effective in managing glucose in patients with diabetes on enteral nutrition.

Author Contributions: Both authors contributed significantly in all aspects of the manuscript. They read and approved the final copy.

Conflicts of Interest: The authors declare no conflict of interest.

References

1. Ojo, O. Diabetes in ethnic minorities in UK: The role of diet in glucose dysregulation and prevalence of diabetes. *J. Food Nutr. Disord.* **2013**, *2*, 1–7.
2. Ojo, O. The impact of changes in health and social care on enteral feeding in the community. *Nutrients* **2012**, *4*, 1709–1722. [CrossRef] [PubMed]
3. Hanif, M.W.; Valsamakis, G.; Dixon, A.; Boutsiadis, A.; Jones, A.F.; Barnett, A.H.; Kumar, S. Detection of impaired glucose tolerance and undiagnosed type 2 diabetes in UK South Asians: An effective screening strategy. *Diabetes Obes. Metab.* **2008**, *10*, 755–762. [CrossRef] [PubMed]
4. Polikandrioti, M.; Dokoutsidou, H. The role of exercise and nutrition in type 2 diabetes mellitus management. *Health Sci. J.* **2009**, *3*, 216–221.
5. Ojo, O. Balloon gastrostomy tubes for long-term feeding in the community. *Br. J. Nurs.* **2011**, *20*, 34–38. [CrossRef] [PubMed]
6. Ojo, O. Managing patients on enteral feeding tubes in the community. *Br. J. Community Nurs.* **2010**, *15*, 6–13. [CrossRef] [PubMed]
7. Lubart, E.; Segal, R.; Wainstein, J.; Marinov, G.; Yarovoy, A.; Leibovitz, A. Evaluation of an intra-institutional diabetes disease management programme for the glycaemic control of elderly long-term diabetic patients. *Geriatr. Gerontol. Int.* **2014**, *14*, 341–345. [CrossRef] [PubMed]
8. Ojo, O. Evaluating care: Home enteral nutrition. *J. Community Nurs.* **2010**, *24*, 18–25.
9. Ojo, O.; Patel, I. Home enteral nutrition and team working. *J. Community Nurs.* **2012**, *26*, 15–18.
10. Vindedzis, S.A.; Marsh, B.; Sherriff, J.L.; Stanton, K.G. Hypoglycaemia in inpatients with diabetes on nasogastric feeding. *Pract. Diabetes* **2014**, *31*, 29–31.
11. Ojo, O.; Bowden, J. Infection control in enteral feed and feeding systems in the community. *Br. J. Nurs.* **2012**, *21*, 1070–1075. [CrossRef] [PubMed]
12. Pohl, M.; Mayr, P.; Mertl-Roetzer, M.; Lauster, F.; Haslbeck, M.; Hipper, B.; Steube, D.; Tietjen, M.; Eriksen, J.; Rahlfs, V.W. Glycaemic control in patients with type 2 diabetes mellitus with a disease specific enteral formula: Stage II of a randomised controlled multicentre trial. *J. Parenter. Enter. Nutr.* **2009**, *33*, 37–49. [CrossRef]
13. Ojo, O. Managing Diabetes in people on home enteral tube feeding. *Diabetes Prim. Care* **2012**, *14*, 113–119.
14. Ojo, O. Problems with use of a Foley catheter in home enteral tube feeding. *Br. J. Nurs.* **2014**, *23*, 360–364. [CrossRef] [PubMed]
15. González Infantino, C.A.; González, C.D.; Sánchez, R.; Presner, N. Hyperglycaemia and hypoalbuminemia as prognostic mortality factors in patients with enteral feeding. *Nutrition* **2013**, *29*, 497–501. [CrossRef] [PubMed]
16. Cortinovis, F.; Cortesi, L.; Sileo, F. Protocol for blood glucose control during enteral nutrition induction in patients with diabetes mellitus. *Mediterr. J. Nutr. Metab.* **2009**, *1*, 159–163. [CrossRef]

17. Qaseem, A.; Chou, R.; Humphrey, L.L.; Shekelle, P. Inpatient glycaemic control: Best practice advice from the clinical guidelines committee of the American College of Physicians. *Am. J. Med. Qual.* **2014**, *29*. [CrossRef]

18. Wright, K.; Ojo, O. Foot care for residents with type 2 diabetes. *Nurs. Resid. Care* **2010**, *12*, 585–589.

19. Elia, M.; Ceriello, A.; Laube, H.; Sinclair, A.J.; Engfer, M.; Stratton, R.J. Enteral nutritional support and use of diabetes specific formulas for patients with diabetes. *Diabetes Care* **2005**, *28*, 2267–2279. [CrossRef] [PubMed]

20. National Collaborating Centre for Chronic Conditions. *Type 2 diabetes: National Clinical Guideline for Management in Primary and Secondary Care (Update)*; Royal College of Physicians: London, UK, 2008.

21. Ceriello, A.; Lansink, M.; Rouws, C.H.F.C.; van Laere, K.M.J.; Frost, G.S. Administration of a new diabetes specific enteral formula results in an improved 24 h glucose profile in type 2 diabetic patients. *Diabetes Res. Clin. Pract.* **2009**, *84*, 259–266. [CrossRef] [PubMed]

22. Hise, M.E.; Fuhrman, M.P. *The Effect of Diabetes Specific Enteral Formulae on Clinical and Glycaemic Indicators*; Parrish, C.R., Ed.; Nutrition Issues in Gastroenterology Series 74; Shugar Publishing: New York, NY, USA, 2009; pp. 20–36.

23. McMahon, M.M.; Nystrom, E.; Braunschweig, C.; Miles, J.; Compher, C. The American Society of Parenteral and Enteral Nutrition (ASPEN) Clinical Guidelines: Nutrition support of adult patients with hyperglycaemia. *J. Parenter. Enter. Nutr.* **2013**, *37*, 23–36. [CrossRef]

24. Cheng, A.Y.Y. Achieving glycaemic control in special populations in hospital: Perspectives in practice. *Can. J. Diabetes* **2014**, *38*, 134–138. [CrossRef] [PubMed]

25. Bettany-Saltikov, J. *How to Do a Systematic Literature Review in Nursing*; Ashford Colour Press Ltd.: Gosport, Hampshire, UK, 2012.

26. Wright, R.W.; Brand, R.A.; Dunn, W.; Spindler, K.P. How to write a systematic review. *Clin. Orthop. Relat. Res.* **2007**, *455*, 23–29. [CrossRef] [PubMed]

27. Alish, C.J.; Garvey, W.T.; Maki, K.C.; Sacks, G.S.; Hustead, D.S.; Hegazi, R.A.; Mustad, V.A. A diabetes specific enteral formula improves glycaemic variability in patients with type 2 diabetes. *Diabetes Technol. Ther.* **2010**, *12*, 419–425. [CrossRef] [PubMed]

28. Vaisman, N.; Lansink, M.; Rouws, C.H.; van Laere, K.M.; Segal, R.; Niv, E.; Bowling, T.E.; Waitzberg, D.L.; Morley, J.E. Tube feeding with a diabetes specific feed for 12 weeks improves glycaemic control in type 2 diabetes patients. *Clin. Nutr.* **2009**, *28*, 549–555. [CrossRef] [PubMed]

29. Voss, A.C.; Maki, K.C.; Garvey, W.T.; Hustead, D.S.; Alish, C.; Fix, B.; Mustad, V.A. Effect of two carbohydrate modified tube feeding formulas on metabolic responses in patients with type 2 diabetes. *Nutrition* **2008**, *24*, 990–997. [CrossRef] [PubMed]

30. De Luis, D.A.; Izaola, O.; Aller, R.; Cuellar, L.; Terroba, M.C.; Martin, T.; Cabezas, G.; Rojo, S.; Domingo, M. A randomised clinical trial with two enteral diabetes specific supplements in patients with diabetes mellitus type 2: Metabolic effects. *Eur. Rev. Med. Pharmacol. Sci.* **2008**, *12*, 261–266. [PubMed]

31. Hofman, Z.; van Drunen, J.D.E.; de Later, C.; Kuipers, H. The effect of different nutritional feeds on the postprandial glucose response in healthy volunteers and patients with type 2 diabetes. *Eur. J. Clin. Nutr.* **2004**, *58*, 1553–1556. [CrossRef] [PubMed]

32. Hofman, Z.; van Drunen, J.D.E.; de Later, C.; Kuipers, H. The Glycaemic index of standard and diabetes specific enteral formulas. *Asia Pac. J. Clin. Nutr.* **2006**, *15*, 412–417. [PubMed]

33. Hassan, A.; Elobeid, T.; Kerkadi, A.; Medhat, M.; Suheil, G. Glycaemic index of selected carbohydrate based foods consumed in Qatar. *Int. J. Food Sci. Nutr.* **2010**, *61*, 512–518. [CrossRef] [PubMed]

34. Charney, P.; Hertzler, S.R. Management of blood glucose and diabetes in the critically ill patient receiving enteral feeding. *Nutr. Clin. Pract.* **2004**, *19*, 129–136. [CrossRef] [PubMed]

35. Via, M.A.; Mechanick, J.I. Inpatient enteral and parenteral nutrition for patients with diabetes. *Curr. Diab. Rep.* **2011**, *11*, 99–105. [CrossRef] [PubMed]

36. Widanagamage, R.D.; Ekanayake, S.; Welihinda, J. Carbohydrate-rich foods: Glycaemic indices and the effect of constituent macronutrients. *Int. J. Food Sci. Nutr.* **2009**, *60*, 215–223. [CrossRef] [PubMed]

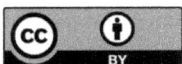

nutrients

MDPI

Review

Microbiome Associations of Therapeutic Enteral Nutrition

Rajesh Shah [1] and Richard Kellermayer [2,*]

[1] Department of Internal Medicine, Section of Gastroenterology, Baylor College of Medicine, Houston, TX, 77030, USA; rajeshs@bcm.edu

[2] Department of Pediatrics, Section of Gastroenterology, Baylor College of Medicine and Texas Children's Hospital, Houston, TX, 77030, USA

* Author to whom correspondence should be addressed; kellerma@bcm.edu; Tel.: +1-832-822-1051; Fax: +1-832-825-3633.

Received: 21 August 2014; in revised form: 8 October 2014; Accepted: 21 October 2014; Published: 21 November 2014

Abstract: One of the most effective forms of therapeutic enteral nutrition is designated as "exclusive enteral nutrition" (EEN). EEN constitutes the monotonous enteral delivery of complete liquid nutrition and has been most explored in the treatment Crohn's disease (CD), a form of inflammatory bowel disease. While EEN's mechanisms of action are not clearly understood, it has been shown to modify the composition of the intestinal microbiome, an important component of CD pathogenesis. The current literature on the intestinal microbiome in healthy individuals and CD patients is reviewed with respect to EEN therapy. Further investigations in this field are needed to better understand the role and potential for EEN in chronic human disorders.

Keywords: enteral nutrition; Crohn's disease; microbiota; IBD; rheumatoid arthritis

1. Introduction

Therapeutic enteral nutrition describes the provision of defined nutritional support with the goal of treating a disease state. Despite a long history using therapeutic enteral nutrition, the critical mechanisms of action by which dietary changes can exert beneficial effects in specific human disorders are incompletely understood. Multiple hypotheses have been put forward in this regard, which include reduction in antigen exposure, overall nutritional repletion, improvement in intestinal barrier function, provision of micronutrients and reduction in dietary fat or carbohydrate, leading to reduced byproducts producing inflammation [1,2].

Exclusive enteral nutrition (EEN) is a subtype of therapeutic nutrition where dietary intake is confined to the persistent delivery of the same complete food preparation. Most commonly, EEN is achieved by liquid enteral formulas. Liquid formulations of EEN are typically divided into either being elemental or polymeric. Elemental formulas deliver a protein source as individual amino acids, and polymeric formulas provide intact protein. EEN has been most commonly employed to treat Crohn's disease (CD) [3]. CD is an incurable subtype of inflammatory bowel diseases (IBDs) characterized by transmural inflammation of the intestine anywhere from the mouth to the anus. The pathogenesis of CD is believed to involve the interaction between a defective intestinal barrier, environmental risk factors, the intestinal microbiome and host genetics [4,5]. Many of these biological systems, apart from genetics, are suspected to be modulated by EEN [2], which may explain its efficacy in treating CD. More recently, the microbiome related effects of this therapeutic nutrition are coming into focus. EEN has also been explored in the treatment of other autoimmune diseases, such as juvenile idiopathic arthritis [6] and ulcerative colitis [7], but these studies are rather limited. Therefore, this review will focus on CD with respect to the microbiome-related influences of EEN.

2. Treatment of CD with EEN

Induction and maintenance of remission (symptom free disease) are the current treatment goals for CD. The available medical therapies to achieve these goals include 5-aminosalicyclic acid (5-ASA) derivatives, immunosuppressive or immunomodulator agents (azathioprine, methotrexate), biologic medications (molecularly-engineered antibodies against key components of the human intestinal inflammatory cascade: infliximab, adalimumab, certolizumab, natalizumab, vedolizumab, *etc.*) or steroids (prednisone, budesonide). For severe CD, induction is typically achievable with either biologics or steroids. Thereafter, the continuation or transition to immunomodulators or biologic agents can substantiate remission. This approach, however, has limitations, including increased risk of adverse events (pancreatitis, hepatitis, neutropenia/bone marrow suppression) and potential long-term complications, such as a higher risk of malignancies [8,9]. Secondary to the limitations of conventional medical treatments, EEN has been explored as an adjunct or monotherapy for CD.

Since steroids are commonly used to induce remission, studies compared the efficacy of EEN to steroids during early CD treatment. Small, randomized trials found that children treated with elemental nutrition or steroids had similar rates of clinical improvement. Elemental EEN, however, was superior to steroids in terms of improved growth velocity [10,11]. Though these results were encouraging, the treatment durations were only 4–6 weeks, leaving questions about the potential for EEN as a maintenance therapy. Another limitation of these studies was non-compliance, since 8%–11% of children were unable to tolerate the elemental diet due to bad taste.

To overcome the limitations of elemental EEN, some trials have used polymeric formulas to induce or maintain remission in CD patients. Early investigations comparing polymeric formulations to steroids suggested that steroids were superior for inducing remission [12,13]; however, more recent work demonstrated equal efficacy of the two treatments [14,15]. Comparison between these trials is difficult, since they used different formulations of polymeric nutrition and for varied durations. Small cohort studies have examined if patients maintained on EEN (elemental or polymeric) remain in remission, but the results suggested that approximately 40%–60% will relapse within a year [16–18]. However, a significant proportion of this relapse rate may be attributed to discontinuation of EEN, which occurred in 20%–50% of the patients. These studies indicate that elemental and polymeric nutrition have equal therapeutic efficacy in CD, so either may be considered. Despite encouraging efficacy results for polymeric nutrition, high relapse rates likely arising from patient non-compliance and deliberate discontinuation due to taste limit EEN as a maintenance therapy for CD.

The discussed studies predominantly used clinical scores (Crohn's Disease Activity Index, CDAI) to determine treatment efficiency. More recently, the demonstration of intestinal mucosal healing is becoming a favored treatment endpoint [19]. Mucosal healing has been correlated with reduced risk of disease relapse, for example [20]. Steroids do not effectively induce mucosal healing, but several studies have shown that EEN can [21–24]. Borrelli *et al.* demonstrated in a randomized controlled trial of 37 children with CD that EEN induced mucosal healing in a greater proportion of patients compared to corticosteroids ($p < 0.001$) at 10 weeks. A single small cohort trial observed that polymeric nutrition induced mucosal healing by magnetic resonance enterography imaging [25]. Magnetic resonance enterography (MRE) can noninvasively detect small bowel mucosal damage with a high sensitivity [26,27]. These studies suggest that EEN may be an efficacious therapy for healing mucosal injury related to CD, but definitive conclusions are limited by patients frequently receiving concomitant IBD medications (6-mercaptopurine, mesalamine, *etc.*). Further well-designed studies will be needed to confirm these findings while controlling for other confounding factors.

Based on the above, EEN appears to be as efficacious and perhaps even superior to steroids, for inducing remission in CD. EEN has several other benefits compared to steroids, including improved growth [10,11] and quality of life [28], optimized bone metabolism [29] and induction of mucosal healing [21–23]. Another common complication of CD is intestinal stricturing, which can necessitate intestinal resections. The risk of recurrence and subsequent surgeries remains high after resections [30]. Interestingly, a recent prospective cohort study from Japan indicated that even partial (50% caloric requirements) delivery of EEN can significantly reduce the endoscopic (mucosal) recurrence of the disease at the surgical site after a year of surgery [31]. The overall need for re-operation tended to be less as well ($p = 0.08$) in the partially EEN-treated group.

Despite the encouraging findings above, EEN has to be further explored to clearly determine its therapeutic potential as an induction and/or maintenance therapy for CD. The questions of its utility as a mono- *versus* combination therapy and as exclusive *versus* partial nutrition remain to be answered, as well. Community-based data from Spain suggested that physicians are frequently (63%) recommending EEN to CD patients [32], but several barriers (poor long-term compliance, lack of optimized teaching, variable patient acceptance) create practical limitations for exploring the full potential of this promising treatment modality. Additionally, the mechanism of action for EEN would be important to define for the optimization of this practically challenging treatment, which carries a desirable side effect spectrum, compared to other available medical therapies. In the next section, we will review our limited understanding of EEN biology.

3. EEN Mechanisms of Action

Several hypotheses have been proposed to explain the efficacy of EEN for CD. The most likely mechanisms include direct anti-inflammatory effects, improvement of intestinal barrier function and modulation of the intestinal microbiome (Figure 1).

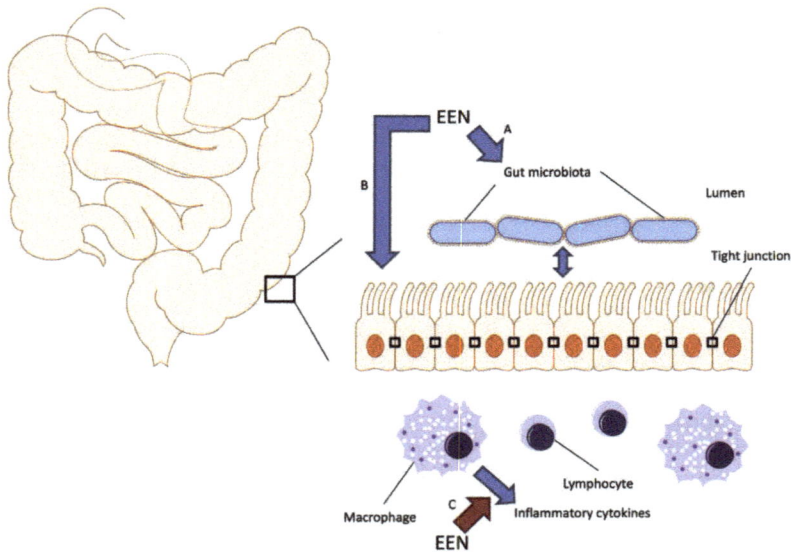

Figure 1. Schematic representation of the gut microbiota, the intestinal epithelium and immune system; and how exclusive enteral nutrition (EEN) may affect these systems. Crohn's disease is associated with dysbiosis of the gut microbiota, increased permeability of the intestinal epithelium and dysregulated immunity. Studies suggest that EEN can alter the composition of the gut microbiota (A), reduce intestinal permeability through modulation of tight junctions either directly (B) or through modulating the intestinal microbiome (A) and downregulate the production of inflammatory cytokines either directly (C) or through modulating the intestinal microbiome (A).

CD is characterized by increased production of multiple pro-inflammatory cytokines (TNF-alpha, IL-1, IL-6, *etc.*) [33]. Studies in children have shown that treatment with polymeric enteral nutrition can downregulate mucosal concentrations of these cytokines, as well as improve mucosal integrity [34].

Similar results were found using *in vitro* techniques, where pro-inflammatory signaling pathways were downregulated in the presence of polymeric formula [35,36]. These studies, however, were limited, since a precise molecular mechanism could not be defined, and the authors acknowledged the need for further work in this area.

Mucosal barrier integrity is vital to the proper functioning of the intestines. Mucosal barrier function is maintained in part by structures designated as tight junctions, which join epithelial cells and participate in the regulation of ion, nutrient and water transport. In CD, the mucosal barrier is dysfunctional, which can be beneficially modified with EEN [37]. *In vitro* models using colonic epithelial cells have demonstrated that EEN can reduce intestinal permeability after the induction of colitis [38,39]. Interestingly, clinical studies have also shown that first-degree family members of CD patients have increased intestinal mucosal permeability when compared to non-IBD controls [40]. These findings suggest that patients with CD have intrinsic mucosal barrier defects, which could be modulated by EEN. However, the exact means by which EEN may improve mucosal permeability are not well understood.

Recent advances in sequencing technologies and bioinformatics have also allowed for examining the potential influence of EEN on the intestinal microbiome, which is another critically important biological system in the pathogenesis of CD. We will next review the human gut microbiome and its potential importance in CD and EEN therapy.

4. Microbiome Basics

The human intestinal microbiome comprises a diverse, highly-interactive ecological system of bacteria, Archaea, viruses and fungi [41]. Classically, the intestinal microbiome was characterized by standard microbiological techniques, but those were inherently limited by the inability to culture over 60% of intestinal bacteria. Recently, investigators have leveraged the conserved 16S rRNA gene present in all bacteria to characterize the intestinal microbiome with sequencing techniques. This gene has taxon-specific variable regions, the sequencing of which can allow for bacterial classification. Additional techniques have been developed to sequence all genes present in a tissue sample (whole genome sequencing, WGS) and characterize the overall gene content attributed to microbes [42,43]. These techniques allow for bacterial classification and examination of overall gene content, but lack the ability to provide information about the actual biological activity or function of a specific microbiome. The functional activity of microbiomes is more specifically examined by the maturing fields of metatranscriptomics and metabolomics [42,44].

In parallel with the application of these new sequencing techniques, bioinformatic tools have been developed to process and interpret large datasets [42,45,46]. These tools enable the generation of common ecological measures (richness and diversity) to characterize the intestinal microbiome community. Richness describes the number of unique bacterial (or other microbial) species present in a sample, and diversity accounts for both the number and the relative abundance of the different species. As microbial clinical studies incorporate these metrics, investigators are finding significant associations with multiple diseases, such as obesity [47] and IBD [48].

Results from the American Human Microbiome Project (HMP) and European metagenomics of the human intestinal tract (MetaHIT) projects have provided composition and functional information for the healthy human microbiome [49,50]. These studies showed highly varying intestinal microbiome composition between subjects, but an overall similar functional capacity. From these and subsequent work, we gained an appreciation for the multitude of factors influencing microbiome composition (age, diet, sampling method). Microbiome composition appears to fluctuate rapidly early in life, remain relatively stable during adulthood and change again towards the seventh decade of life [41]. In addition to age, long-term dietary patterns strongly influence the intestinal microbiome [51–53]. Additionally, the intestinal microbiome can rapidly respond to short-term dietary interventions, as well, but reverts to its prior composition once the interventions cease [54–56]. Furthermore, the gut microbiome is different at the mucosal surface from that of luminal content. Therefore, the clinical sample type (feces *versus* mucosa) has to be taken into consideration [57,58], when planning and comparing microbiome studies of the gut specifically.

5. EEN Effects on the Intestinal Microbiome

A limited number of studies have described the intestinal microbiome of healthy subjects during EEN. Using a cross-over design, Whelan *et al.* examined the effect of fructooligosaccharide and fiber supplemented EEN on intestinal microbiota. They found that total intestinal bacterial counts were reduced during EEN [59]. However, this work utilized fluorescent *in situ* hybridization (FISH) techniques, which carry significant limitations compared to the current high-throughput technologies. Subsequently, the same group re-analyzed this data to describe the change in *Faecalibacterium prausnitzii* during EEN. *F. prausnitzii* is a commensal, Gram-positive bacterium with anti-inflammatory properties, which has been implicated in CD pathogenesis [60]. Their group found significant reductions in *F. prausnitzii* abundance during fiber supplementation, which demonstrated that diet can modulate specific bacterial concentrations [61]. Associations between *F. prausnitzii*, CD and EEN will be discussed in detail in the subsequent sections.

After characterizing the healthy human microbiome by state-of-the-art technology, investigators are now exploring the differences present in diseases. The term dysbiosis refers to the abnormal composition of the intestinal microbiome and has been studied in multiple disease states (obesity, diabetes, *etc.*). Reduced fecal microbiome richness [47] and diversity [62] were found in obese individuals. WGS revealed compositional differences between those with type 2 diabetes and non-diabetic controls, which may influence overall insulin resistance [63,64]. These and many other association studies indicate that abnormal composition and subsequent pathologic functioning of the microbiome may contribute to human disease.

6. The Gut Microbiome of Crohn's Disease

The intestinal microbiome of CD patients has been found to have overall dysbiosis compared to the datasets from HMP and MetaHIT [65,66]. Hansen *et al.* studied colon biopsy specimens from treatment-naive pediatric CD patients and detected significant reductions in diversity compared to healthy controls and patients with ulcerative colitis (UC, the other form of IBD) [65]. Gevers and colleagues examined both stool and mucosal samples from a very large cohort of treatment-naive pediatric CD patients and found modest overall differences compared to controls, which was increased in patients with higher disease activity (Table 1) [66]. Detailed bioinformatic analyses revealed further functional differences between CD and controls. CD microbiomes expressed pathways involved in inflammation and had reduced functionality related to amino acid, carbohydrate and nucleotide metabolism [66]. Other investigations in treatment-experienced CD patients have identified similar functional changes [67,68].

Table 1. Description of mucosal microbiota changes found in treatment-naive Crohn's disease [65, 66]. Several bacterial taxa are increased or decreased compared to non-IBD controls. * Changes in *Faecalibacterium* were inconsistent across studies, with one study reporting an increase and the other a decrease.

Crohn's Disease	
Increased	**Decreased**
Enterobacteriaceae	Bacteroidales
Pasteurellaceae	Clostridiales
Fusobacteriaceae	*Erysipelotrichaceae*
Neisseriaceae	*Bifidobacteriaceae*
Veillonellaceae	*Coriobacteriaceae*
Gemellaceae	*Faecalibacterium* *
Faecalibacterium	

The role of specific bacteria in CD is less understood. The difficulties in making a definite conclusion about single species are well demonstrated by the example of *F. prausnitzii*. Previous observations noted reduced concentrations of *F. prausnitzii* in the terminal ileum of CD patients and higher concentrations correlated with reduced risk of recurrence [69,70]. These studies, however, were confounded by examining treatment-experienced patients, where microbiome composition may have been modified by the treatments themselves [67,71]. Explorations in treatment-naive patients led to conflicting results on *F. prausnitzii*, with one small cohort reporting higher abundance of the bacterium compared to controls [65], as opposed to a lower abundance found in a recent large-scale study [66].

These studies emphasize the complexity of the microbiome in IBD and underscore the need for careful planning (*i.e.*, accounting for confounding factors, recruiting adequate number of patients) to enable the detection of meaningful differences. These limitations have to be taken into account when interpreting the available literature on EEN-microbiome effects in CD patients.

7. EEN Induced Microbiome Changes in CD Patients

Only a few studies have examined the microbial effects of EEN in CD patients. Lionetti *et al.* reported results from a small case series of nine pediatric CD patients treated with polymeric enteral nutrition. They noted that eight of nine children obtained clinical remission, and all experienced significant shifts in intestinal microbiome composition [72]. These shifts were determined using the gel electrophoresis banding pattern, resulting in a limited depth of interrogation when compared to high-throughput technologies. Similar results were found in a study of six children with CD treated with EEN, as well as correlations between specific bacterial taxa and the degree of inflammation [73]. In a recently published work on EEN treatment for pediatric CD (utilizing gel electrophoresis and quantitative real-time PCR), investigators found decreases in overall microbiome diversity and reductions in *F. prausnitzii* abundance during EEN therapy [74]. These findings challenge the previous notions of increased microbiome diversity associated with health and higher concentrations of *F. prausnitzii* associated with reduced CD activity. In accordance with the difficulties for interpreting the role of *F. prausnitzii* in CD, some observations indicate that regardless of disease activity, the abundance of it remains low in CD [75] and can even further decrease upon clinical improvement with elemental enteral therapy [76]. Clearly, further work is required to understand the role of *F. prausnitzii* in CD and IBD in general. Such controversies emphasize the challenges of microbiome research, even in the current era of advanced technology.

To gain a better understanding of EEN's effects on the intestinal microbiome, our lab explored this interaction in a mouse model. We set up the hypothesis that it is the monotonous nature of EEN that is critical to its therapeutic effect and not the liquid nature or low antigenicity of it. Healthy mice were assigned to either a single chow or alternating chows. This was meant to mimic either EEN or a more free (liberalized) diet, respectively. After 20 days of the monotonous or the alternating diet feeding, mice were given dextran sulfate sodium (DSS), an intestinal irritant that induces acute large bowel inflammation (colitis) and is an accepted model of human IBD. Mice given the single chow diets, similar to EEN, had higher overall microbiome diversity compared to alternating chow fed mice [77]. These results were consistent with the prior human findings described by Leach *et al.* [73]. However, the results of Gerasimidis and colleagues [74] oppose the observations in the murine experiment. Regardless, the mice provided alternating chow were also more susceptible to intestinal injury from DSS, supporting an association between reduced microbiome diversity and susceptibility to colitis in mammals. This observation is also consistent with the reduction of microbiome diversity in IBD patients [65,66]. Altogether, our murine model work supported the hypothesis that the monotonous nature of EEN may be a key component to its efficacy. Epidemiologic observations correlating agricultural import with the incidence of CD in a European country further substantiated the possible validity of the "monotonous diet" hypothesis [77]. Further high-throughput studies will need to explore the effects of EEN on microbiome composition in both healthy people and CD patients to elucidate the exact effects of this nutritional therapy in health and disease.

8. Future Considerations and Conclusions

Several randomized clinical trials have shown the efficacy for partial and exclusive elemental or polymeric nutritional therapies to induce clinical improvement and even remission in CD. EEN appears to be superior to steroids with respect to the induction of mucosal healing during induction therapy and may have the potential to provide long-term remission in some cases of CD. The highlighted limitations of the existing clinical studies and the practical challenges for this drastic nutritional therapy warrant further intense work towards the optimization of this treatment modality. Though the mechanism(s) of action of nutritional therapy remains unknown, the detected changes in the intestinal microbiome composition and function induced by EEN provide new routes for research. The findings from such investigations may facilitate the development of novel treatment strategies, not only for CD, but for other autoimmune disorders, as well.

Acknowledgments: The authors would like to thank the Gutsy Kids Fund, including philanthropic donation from the Karen and Brock Wagner family and other generous families.

Author Contributions: Rajesh Shah: conception, drafting and editing of the manuscript; Richard Kellermayer: conception, drafting, editing and final approval of the manuscript.

Conflicts of Interest: The authors declare no conflict of interest.

References

1. Critch, J.; Day, A.S.; Otley, A.; King-Moore, C.; Teitelbaum, J.E.; Shashidhar, H.; Committee, N.I. Use of enteral nutrition for the control of intestinal inflammation in pediatric Crohn disease. *J. Pediatr. Gastroenterol. Nutr.* **2012**, *54*, 298–305. [CrossRef] [PubMed]

2. Nahidi, L.; Day, A.S.; Lemberg, D.A.; Leach, S.T. Paediatric inflammatory bowel disease: A mechanistic approach to investigate exclusive enteral nutrition treatment. *Scientifica* **2014**, *2014*. [CrossRef]

3. Zachos, M.; Tondeur, M.; Griffiths, A.M. Enteral nutritional therapy for induction of remission in Crohn's disease. *Cochrane Database Syst. Rev.* **2007**, *1*. [CrossRef]

4. Xavier, R.J.; Podolsky, D.K. Unravelling the pathogenesis of inflammatory bowel disease. *Nature* **2007**, *448*, 427–434. [CrossRef] [PubMed]

5. Kellermayer, R. Epigenetics and the developmental origins of inflammatory bowel diseases. *Can. J. Gastroenterol.* **2012**, *26*, 909–915. [PubMed]

6. Berntson, L. Anti-inflammatory effect by exclusive enteral nutrition (EEN) in a patient with juvenile idiopathic arthritis (JIA): Brief report. *Clin. Rheumatol.* **2014**, *33*, 1173–1175. [CrossRef] [PubMed]

7. González-Huix, F.; Fernández-Bañares, F.; Esteve-Comas, M.; Abad-Lacruz, A.; Cabré, E.; Acero, D.; Figa, M.; Guilera, M.; Humbert, P.; de León, R.; *et al.* Enteral *versus* parenteral nutrition as adjunct therapy in acute ulcerative colitis. *Am. J. Gastroenterol.* **1993**, *88*, 227–232.

8. Siegel, C.A.; Marden, S.M.; Persing, S.M.; Larson, R.J.; Sands, B.E. Risk of lymphoma associated with combination anti-tumor necrosis factor and immunomodulator therapy for the treatment of Crohn's disease: A meta-analysis. *Clin. Gastroenterol. Hepatol. Off. Clin. Pract. J. Am. Gastroenterol. Assoc.* **2009**, *7*, 874–881.

9. Long, M.D.; Martin, C.F.; Pipkin, C.A.; Herfarth, H.H.; Sandler, R.S.; Kappelman, M.D. Risk of melanoma and nonmelanoma skin cancer among patients with inflammatory bowel disease. *Gastroenterology* **2012**, *143*, 390–399. [CrossRef] [PubMed]

10. Sanderson, I.R.; Udeen, S.; Davies, P.S.; Savage, M.O.; Walker-Smith, J.A. Remission induced by an elemental diet in small bowel Crohn's disease. *Arch. Dis. Childhood* **1987**, *62*, 123–127. [CrossRef]

11. Thomas, A.G.; Taylor, F.; Miller, V. Dietary intake and nutritional treatment in childhood Crohn's disease. *J. Pediatr. Gastroenterol. Nutr.* **1993**, *17*, 75–81. [CrossRef] [PubMed]

12. Malchow, H.; Steinhardt, H.J.; Lorenz-Meyer, H.; Strohm, W.D.; Rasmussen, S.; Sommer, H.; Jarnum, S.; Brandes, J.W.; Leonhardt, H.; Ewe, K.; *et al.* Feasibility and effectiveness of a defined-formula diet regimen in treating active Crohn's disease. European cooperative Crohn's disease study III. *Scand. J. Gastroenterol.* **1990**, *25*, 235–244.

13. Lochs, H.; Steinhardt, H.J.; Klaus-Wentz, B.; Zeitz, M.; Vogelsang, H.; Sommer, H.; Fleig, W.E.; Bauer, P.; Schirrmeister, J.; Malchow, H. Comparison of enteral nutrition and drug treatment in active Crohn's disease. Results of the european cooperative Crohn's disease study IV. *Gastroenterology* **1991**, *101*, 881–888. [PubMed]

14. Gonzalez-Huix, F.; de Leon, R.; Fernandez-Banares, F.; Esteve, M.; Cabre, E.; Acero, D.; Abad-Lacruz, A.; Figa, M.; Guilera, M.; Planas, R.; *et al.* Polymeric enteral diets as primary treatment of active Crohn's disease: A prospective steroid controlled trial. *Gut* **1993**, *34*, 778–782. [CrossRef]

15. Ruuska, T.; Savilahti, E.; Maki, M.; Ormala, T.; Visakorpi, J.K. Exclusive whole protein enteral diet *versus* prednisolone in the treatment of acute Crohn's disease in children. *J. Pediatr. Gastroenterol. Nutr.* **1994**, *19*, 175–180. [CrossRef]

16. Takagi, S.; Utsunomiya, K.; Kuriyama, S.; Yokoyama, H.; Takahashi, S.; Iwabuchi, M.; Takahashi, H.; Takahashi, S.; Kinouchi, Y.; Hiwatashi, N.; *et al.* Effectiveness of an 'half elemental diet' as maintenance therapy for Crohn's disease: A randomized-controlled trial. *Aliment. Pharmacol. Ther.* **2006**, *24*, 1333–1340. [CrossRef]

17. Duncan, H.; Buchanan, E.; Cardigan, T.; Garrick, V.; Curtis, L.; McGrogan, P.; Barclay, A.; Russell, R.K. A retrospective study showing maintenance treatment options for paediatric Crohn's disease in the first year following diagnosis after induction of remission with EEN: Supplemental enteral nutrition is better than nothing! *BMC Gastroenterol.* **2014**, *14*. [CrossRef]

18. Knight, C.; El-Matary, W.; Spray, C.; Sandhu, B.K. Long-term outcome of nutritional therapy in paediatric Crohn's disease. *Clin. Nutr.* **2005**, *24*, 775–779. [CrossRef] [PubMed]

19. Peyrin-Biroulet, L.; Bressenot, A.; Kampman, W. Histologic remission: The ultimate therapeutic goal in ulcerative colitis? *Clin. Gastroenterol. Hepatol. Off. Clin. Pract. J. Am. Gastroenterol. Assoc.* **2014**, *12*, 929–934.

20. Ardizzone, S.; Cassinotti, A.; Duca, P.; Mazzali, C.; Penati, C.; Manes, G.; Marmo, R.; Massari, A.; Molteni, P.; Maconi, G.; *et al.* Mucosal healing predicts late outcomes after the first course of corticosteroids for newly diagnosed ulcerative colitis. *Clin. Gastroenterol. Hepatol. Off. Clin. Pract. J. Am. Gastroenterol. Assoc.* **2011**, *9*, 483–489.

21. Rubio, A.; Pigneur, B.; Garnier-Lengline, H.; Talbotec, C.; Schmitz, J.; Canioni, D.; Goulet, O.; Ruemmele, F.M. The efficacy of exclusive nutritional therapy in paediatric Crohn's disease, comparing fractionated oral *vs.* Continuous enteral feeding. *Aliment. Pharmacol. Ther.* **2011**, *33*, 1332–1339. [CrossRef]

22. Borrelli, O.; Cordischi, L.; Cirulli, M.; Paganelli, M.; Labalestra, V.; Uccini, S.; Russo, P.M.; Cucchiara, S. Polymeric diet alone *versus* corticosteroids in the treatment of active pediatric Crohn's disease: A randomized controlled open-label trial. *Clin. Gastroenterol. Hepatol. Off. Clin. Pract. J. Am. Gastroenterol Assoc.* **2006**, *4*, 744–753.

23. Berni Canani, R.; Terrin, G.; Borrelli, O.; Romano, M.T.; Manguso, F.; Coruzzo, A.; D'Armiento, F.; Romeo, E.F.; Cucchiara, S. Short- and long-term therapeutic efficacy of nutritional therapy and corticosteroids in paediatric Crohn's disease. *Dig. Liver Dis.* **2006**, *38*, 381–387. [CrossRef]

24. Navas-Lopez, V.M.; Blasco-Alonso, J.; Maseri, S.L.; Giron Fernandez-Crehuet, F.; Serrano Nieto, M.J.; Vicioso Recio, M.I.; Sierra Salinas, C. Exclusive enteral nutrition continues to be first line therapy for pediatric Crohn's disease in the era of biologics. *Anales de Pediatria* **2014**. [CrossRef]

25. Grover, Z.; Muir, R.; Lewindon, P. Exclusive enteral nutrition induces early clinical, mucosal and transmural remission in paediatric Crohn's disease. *J. Gastroenterol.* **2014**, *49*, 638–645. [CrossRef] [PubMed]

26. Qiu, Y.; Mao, R.; Chen, B.L.; Li, X.H.; He, Y.; Zeng, Z.R.; Li, Z.P.; Chen, M.H. Systematic review with meta-analysis: Magnetic resonance enterography *vs.* Computed tomography enterography for evaluating disease activity in small bowel Crohn's disease. *Aliment. Pharmacol. Ther.* **2014**, *40*, 134–146. [CrossRef]

27. Ordas, I.; Rimola, J.; Rodriguez, S.; Paredes, J.M.; Martinez-Perez, M.J.; Blanc, E.; Arevalo, J.A.; Aduna, M.; Andreu, M.; Radosevic, A.; *et al.* Accuracy of magnetic resonance enterography in assessing response to therapy and mucosal healing in patients with Crohn's disease. *Gastroenterology* **2014**, *146*, 374–382. [CrossRef]

28. Afzal, N.A.; van Der Zaag-Loonen, H.J.; Arnaud-Battandier, F.; Davies, S.; Murch, S.; Derkx, B.; Heuschkel, R.; Fell, J.M. Improvement in quality of life of children with acute Crohn's disease does not parallel mucosal healing after treatment with exclusive enteral nutrition. *Aliment. Pharmacol. Ther.* **2004**, *20*, 167–172. [CrossRef] [PubMed]

29. Whitten, K.E.; Leach, S.T.; Bohane, T.D.; Woodhead, H.J.; Day, A.S. Effect of exclusive enteral nutrition on bone turnover in children with Crohn's disease. *J. Gastroenterol.* **2010**, *45*, 399–405. [CrossRef] [PubMed]

30. Van Loo, E.S.; Dijkstra, G.; Ploeg, R.J.; Nieuwenhuijs, V.B. Prevention of postoperative recurrence of Crohn's disease. *J. Crohns Colitis.* **2012**, *6*, 637–646. [CrossRef] [PubMed]

31. Yamamoto, T.; Shiraki, M.; Nakahigashi, M.; Umegae, S.; Matsumoto, K. Enteral nutrition to suppress postoperative Crohn's disease recurrence: A five-year prospective cohort study. *Int. J. Colorect. Dis.* **2013**, *28*, 335–340. [CrossRef]

32. Navas-Lopez, V.M.; Martin-de-Carpi, J.; Segarra, O.; Garcia-Burriel, J.I.; Diaz-Martin, J.J.; Rodriguez, A.; Medina, E.; Juste, M. Present; prescription of enteral nutrition in pediatric Crohn's disease in spain. *Nutric. Hospitalaria* **2014**, *29*, 537–546.

33. Podolsky, D.K. Inflammatory bowel disease. *N. Engl. J. Med.* **2002**, *347*, 417–429. [CrossRef] [PubMed]

34. Fell, J.M.; Paintin, M.; Arnaud-Battandier, F.; Beattie, R.M.; Hollis, A.; Kitching, P.; Donnet-Hughes, A.; MacDonald, T.T.; Walker-Smith, J.A. Mucosal healing and a fall in mucosal pro-inflammatory cytokine mrna induced by a specific oral polymeric diet in paediatric Crohn's disease. *Aliment. Pharmacol. Ther.* **2000**, *14*, 281–289. [CrossRef] [PubMed]

35. De Jong, N.S.; Leach, S.T.; Day, A.S. Polymeric formula has direct anti-inflammatory effects on enterocytes in an *in vitro* model of intestinal inflammation. *Dig. Dis. Sci.* **2007**, *52*, 2029–2036. [CrossRef]

36. Meister, D.; Bode, J.; Shand, A.; Ghosh, S. Anti-inflammatory effects of enteral diet components on Crohn's disease-affected tissues *in vitro*. *Dig. Liver Dis* **2002**, *34*, 430–438. [CrossRef]

37. Edelblum, K.L.; Turner, J.R. The tight junction in inflammatory disease: Communication breakdown. *Curr. Opin. Pharmacol.* **2009**, *9*, 715–720. [CrossRef] [PubMed]

38. Nahidi, L.; Day, A.S.; Lemberg, D.A.; Leach, S.T. Differential effects of nutritional and non-nutritional therapies on intestinal barrier function in an *in vitro* model. *J. Gastroenterol.* **2012**, *47*, 107–117.

39. Nahidi, L.; Leach, S.T.; Mitchell, H.M.; Kaakoush, N.O.; Lemberg, D.A.; Munday, J.S.; Huinao, K.; Day, A.S. Inflammatory bowel disease therapies and gut function in a colitis mouse model. *BioMed. Res. Int.* **2013**, *2013*. [CrossRef] [PubMed]

40. Thjodleifsson, B.; Sigthorsson, G.; Cariglia, N.; Reynisdottir, I.; Gudbjartsson, D.F.; Kristjansson, K.; Meddings, J.B.; Gudnason, V.; Wandall, J.H.; Andersen, L.P.; *et al.* Subclinical intestinal inflammation: An inherited abnormality in Crohn's disease relatives? *Gastroenterology* **2003**, *124*, 1728–1737. [CrossRef] [PubMed]

41. Hollister, E.B.; Gao, C.; Versalovic, J. Compositional and functional features of the gastrointestinal microbiome and their effects on human health. *Gastroenterology* **2014**, *146*, 1449–1458. [CrossRef] [PubMed]

42. Morgan, X.C.; Huttenhower, C. Meta'omic analytic techniques for studying the intestinal microbiome. *Gastroenterology* **2014**, *146*, 1437–1448. [CrossRef] [PubMed]

43. Kuczynski, J.; Lauber, C.L.; Walters, W.A.; Parfrey, L.W.; Clemente, J.C.; Gevers, D.; Knight, R. Experimental and analytical tools for studying the human microbiome. *Nat. Rev. Genet.* **2012**, *13*, 47–58. [CrossRef]

44. Ursell, L.K.; Haiser, H.J.; van Treuren, W.; Garg, N.; Reddivari, L.; Vanamala, J.; Dorrestein, P.C.; Turnbaugh, P.J.; Knight, R. The intestinal metabolome: An intersection between microbiota and host. *Gastroenterology* **2014**, *146*, 1470–1476. [CrossRef] [PubMed]

45. Schloss, P.D.; Westcott, S.L.; Ryabin, T.; Hall, J.R.; Hartmann, M.; Hollister, E.B.; Lesniewski, R.A.; Oakley, B.B.; Parks, D.H.; Robinson, C.J.; *et al.* Introducing mothur: Open-source, platform-independent, community-supported software for describing and comparing microbial communities. *Appl. Environ. Microbiol.* **2009**, *75*, 7537–7541. [CrossRef] [PubMed]

46. Caporaso, J.G.; Kuczynski, J.; Stombaugh, J.; Bittinger, K.; Bushman, F.D.; Costello, E.K.; Fierer, N.; Pena, A.G.; Goodrich, J.K.; Gordon, J.I.; *et al.* Qiime allows analysis of high-throughput community sequencing data. *Nat. Methods* **2010**, *7*, 335–336. [CrossRef] [PubMed]

47. Le Chatelier, E.; Nielsen, T.; Qin, J.; Prifti, E.; Hildebrand, F.; Falony, G.; Almeida, M.; Arumugam, M.; Batto, J.M.; Kennedy, S.; *et al.* Richness of human gut microbiome correlates with metabolic markers. *Nature* **2013**, *500*, 541–546. [CrossRef] [PubMed]

48. Kostic, A.D.; Xavier, R.J.; Gevers, D. The microbiome in inflammatory bowel disease: Current status and the future ahead. *Gastroenterology* **2014**, *146*, 1489–1499. [CrossRef] [PubMed]

49. Human Microbiome Project Consortium. Structure, function and diversity of the healthy human microbiome. *Nature* **2012**, *486*, 207–214.

50. Qin, J.; Li, R.; Raes, J.; Arumugam, M.; Burgdorf, K.S.; Manichanh, C.; Nielsen, T.; Pons, N.; Levenez, F.; Yamada, T.; *et al.* A human gut microbial gene catalogue established by metagenomic sequencing. *Nature* **2010**, *464*, 59–65. [CrossRef] [PubMed]

51. De Filippo, C.; Cavalieri, D.; Di Paola, M.; Ramazzotti, M.; Poullet, J.B.; Massart, S.; Collini, S.; Pieraccini, G.; Lionetti, P. Impact of diet in shaping gut microbiota revealed by a comparative study in children from europe and rural Africa. *Proc. Natl. Acad. Sci. USA* **2010**, *107*, 14691–14696. [CrossRef] [PubMed]

52. Ley, R.E.; Hamady, M.; Lozupone, C.; Turnbaugh, P.J.; Ramey, R.R.; Bircher, J.S.; Schlegel, M.L.; Tucker, T.A.; Schrenzel, M.D.; Knight, R.; *et al.* Evolution of mammals and their gut microbes. *Science* **2008**, *320*, 1647–1651. [CrossRef] [PubMed]

53. Arumugam, M.; Raes, J.; Pelletier, E.; Le Paslier, D.; Yamada, T.; Mende, D.R.; Fernandes, G.R.; Tap, J.; Bruls, T.; Batto, J.M.; *et al.* Enterotypes of the human gut microbiome. *Nature* **2011**, *473*, 174–180. [CrossRef] [PubMed]

54. Cotillard, A.; Kennedy, S.P.; Kong, L.C.; Prifti, E.; Pons, N.; Le Chatelier, E.; Almeida, M.; Quinquis, B.; Levenez, F.; Galleron, N.; *et al.* Dietary intervention impact on gut microbial gene richness. *Nature* **2013**, *500*, 585–588. [CrossRef] [PubMed]

55. Wu, G.D.; Chen, J.; Hoffmann, C.; Bittinger, K.; Chen, Y.Y.; Keilbaugh, S.A.; Bewtra, M.; Knights, D.; Walters, W.A.; Knight, R.; *et al.* Linking long-term dietary patterns with gut microbial enterotypes. *Science* **2011**, *334*, 105–108. [CrossRef] [PubMed]

56. David, L.A.; Maurice, C.F.; Carmody, R.N.; Gootenberg, D.B.; Button, J.E.; Wolfe, B.E.; Ling, A.V.; Devlin, A.S.; Varma, Y.; Fischbach, M.A.; *et al.* Diet rapidly and reproducibly alters the human gut microbiome. *Nature* **2014**, *505*, 559–563. [CrossRef] [PubMed]

57. Zoetendal, E.G.; von Wright, A.; Vilpponen-Salmela, T.; Ben-Amor, K.; Akkermans, A.D.; de Vos, W.M. Mucosa-associated bacteria in the human gastrointestinal tract are uniformly distributed along the colon and differ from the community recovered from feces. *Appl. Environ. Microbiol.* **2002**, *68*, 3401–3407. [CrossRef] [PubMed]

58. Kellermayer, R.; Mir, S.A.; Nagy-Szakal, D.; Cox, S.B.; Dowd, S.E.; Kaplan, J.L.; Sun, Y.; Reddy, S.; Bronsky, J.; Winter, H.S. Microbiota separation and C-reactive protein elevation in treatment-naive pediatric granulomatous Crohn disease. *J. Pediatr. Gastroenterol. Nutr.* **2012**, *55*, 243–250. [CrossRef] [PubMed]

59. Whelan, K.; Judd, P.A.; Preedy, V.R.; Simmering, R.; Jann, A.; Taylor, M.A. Fructooligosaccharides and fiber partially prevent the alterations in fecal microbiota and short-chain fatty acid concentrations caused by standard enteral formula in healthy humans. *J. Nutr.* **2005**, *135*, 1896–1902. [PubMed]

60. Miquel, S.; Martin, R.; Rossi, O.; Bermudez-Humaran, L.G.; Chatel, J.M.; Sokol, H.; Thomas, M.; Wells, J.M.; Langella, P. Faecalibacterium prausnitzii and human intestinal health. *Curr. Opin. Microbiol.* **2013**, *16*, 255–261. [CrossRef] [PubMed]

61. Benus, R.F.; van der Werf, T.S.; Welling, G.W.; Judd, P.A.; Taylor, M.A.; Harmsen, H.J.; Whelan, K. Association between faecalibacterium prausnitzii and dietary fibre in colonic fermentation in healthy human subjects. *Br. J. Nutr.* **2010**, *104*, 693–700. [CrossRef] [PubMed]

62. Turnbaugh, P.J.; Hamady, M.; Yatsunenko, T.; Cantarel, B.L.; Duncan, A.; Ley, R.E.; Sogin, M.L.; Jones, W.J.; Roe, B.A.; Affourtit, J.P.; *et al.* A core gut microbiome in obese and lean twins. *Nature* **2009**, *457*, 480–484. [CrossRef] [PubMed]

63. Karlsson, F.H.; Tremaroli, V.; Nookaew, I.; Bergstrom, G.; Behre, C.J.; Fagerberg, B.; Nielsen, J.; Backhed, F. Gut metagenome in european women with normal, impaired and diabetic glucose control. *Nature* **2013**, *498*, 99–103. [CrossRef] [PubMed]

64. Qin, J.; Li, Y.; Cai, Z.; Li, S.; Zhu, J.; Zhang, F.; Liang, S.; Zhang, W.; Guan, Y.; Shen, D.; *et al.* A metagenome-wide association study of gut microbiota in type 2 diabetes. *Nature* **2012**, *490*, 55–60. [CrossRef] [PubMed]

65. Hansen, R.; Russell, R.K.; Reiff, C.; Louis, P.; McIntosh, F.; Berry, S.H.; Mukhopadhya, I.; Bisset, W.M.; Barclay, A.R.; Bishop, J.; *et al.* Microbiota of de-novo pediatric IBD: Increased faecalibacterium prausnitzii and reduced bacterial diversity in Crohn's but not in ulcerative colitis. *Am. J. Gastroenterol.* **2012**, *107*, 1913–1922. [CrossRef] [PubMed]

66. Gevers, D.; Kugathasan, S.; Denson, L.A.; Vazquez-Baeza, Y.; Van Treuren, W.; Ren, B.; Schwager, E.; Knights, D.; Song, S.J.; Yassour, M.; *et al.* The treatment-naive microbiome in new-onset Crohn's disease. *Cell. Host Microbe* **2014**, *15*, 382–392. [CrossRef] [PubMed]

67. Morgan, X.C.; Tickle, T.L.; Sokol, H.; Gevers, D.; Devaney, K.L.; Ward, D.V.; Reyes, J.A.; Shah, S.A.; LeLeiko, N.; Snapper, S.B.; *et al.* Dysfunction of the intestinal microbiome in inflammatory bowel disease and treatment. *Genome Biol.* **2012**, *13*. [CrossRef]

68. Davenport, M.; Poles, J.; Leung, J.M.; Wolff, M.J.; Abidi, W.M.; Ullman, T.; Mayer, L.; Cho, I.; Loke, P. Metabolic alterations to the mucosal microbiota in inflammatory bowel disease. *Inflamm. Bowel Dis.* **2014**, *20*, 723–731. [CrossRef] [PubMed]

69. Sokol, H.; Pigneur, B.; Watterlot, L.; Lakhdari, O.; Bermudez-Humaran, L.G.; Gratadoux, J.J.; Blugeon, S.; Bridonneau, C.; Furet, J.P.; Corthier, G.; *et al.* Faecalibacterium prausnitzii is an anti-inflammatory commensal bacterium identified by gut microbiota analysis of crohn disease patients. *Proc. Natl. Acad. Sci. USA* **2008**, *105*, 16731–16736. [CrossRef] [PubMed]

70. Rajca, S.; Grondin, V.; Louis, E.; Vernier-Massouille, G.; Grimaud, J.C.; Bouhnik, Y.; Laharie, D.; Dupas, J.L.; Pillant, H.; Picon, L.; *et al.* Alterations in the intestinal microbiome (dysbiosis) as a predictor of relapse after infliximab withdrawal in Crohn's disease. *Inflamm. Bowel Dis.* **2014**, *20*, 978–986. [PubMed]

71. Wills, E.S.; Jonkers, D.M.; Savelkoul, P.H.; Masclee, A.A.; Pierik, M.J.; Penders, J. Fecal microbial composition of ulcerative colitis and Crohn's disease patients in remission and subsequent exacerbation. *PLoS One* **2014**, *9*. [CrossRef] [PubMed]

72. Lionetti, P.; Callegari, M.L.; Ferrari, S.; Cavicchi, M.C.; Pozzi, E.; de Martino, M.; Morelli, L. Enteral nutrition and microflora in pediatric Crohn's disease. *JPEN. J. Parenter. Enter. Nutr.* **2005**, *29* (Suppl. 4), 173–178. [CrossRef]

73. Leach, S.T.; Mitchell, H.M.; Eng, W.R.; Zhang, L.; Day, A.S. Sustained modulation of intestinal bacteria by exclusive enteral nutrition used to treat children with Crohn's disease. *Aliment. Pharmacol. Ther.* **2008**, *28*, 724–733. [CrossRef] [PubMed]

74. Gerasimidis, K.; Bertz, M.; Hanske, L.; Junick, J.; Biskou, O.; Aguilera, M.; Garrick, V.; Russell, R.K.; Blaut, M.; McGrogan, P.; *et al.* Decline in presumptively protective gut bacterial species and metabolites are paradoxically associated with disease improvement in pediatric Crohn's disease during enteral nutrition. *Inflamm. Bowel Dis.* **2014**, *20*, 861–871. [CrossRef] [PubMed]

75. Schwiertz, A.; Jacobi, M.; Frick, J.S.; Richter, M.; Rusch, K.; Kohler, H. Microbiota in pediatric inflammatory bowel disease. *J. Pediatr.* **2010**, *157*, 240–244. [CrossRef] [PubMed]

76. Jia, W.; Whitehead, R.N.; Griffiths, L.; Dawson, C.; Waring, R.H.; Ramsden, D.B.; Hunter, J.O.; Cole, J.A. Is the abundance of Faecalibacterium prausnitzii relevant to Crohn's disease? *FEMS Microbiol. Lett.* **2010**, *310*, 138–144. [CrossRef] [PubMed]

77. Nagy-Szakal, D.; Mir, S.A.; Ross, M.C.; Tatevian, N.; Petrosino, J.F.; Kellermayer, R. Monotonous diets protect against acute colitis in mice: Epidemiologic and therapeutic implications. *J. Pediatr. Gastroenterol. Nutr.* **2013**, *56*, 544–550. [CrossRef] [PubMed]

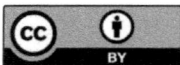

nutrients

MDPI

Review

Nutritional Interventions in Head and Neck Cancer Patients Undergoing Chemoradiotherapy: A Narrative Review

Maurizio Bossola

Department of Surgery, Catholic University, University Hospital "A. Gemelli", Largo A. Gemelli, 8-00168 Rome, Italy; maubosso@tin.it; Tel.: +39-6-30155485; Fax: +39-6-30155491

Received: 10 November 2014; Accepted: 24 December 2014; Published: 5 January 2015

Abstract: The present review aimed to define the role of nutritional interventions in the prevention and treatment of malnutrition in HNC patients undergoing CRT as well as their impact on CRT-related toxicity and survival. Head and neck cancer patients are frequently malnourished at the time of diagnosis and prior to the beginning of treatment. In addition, chemo-radiotherapy (CRT) causes or exacerbates symptoms, such as alteration or loss of taste, mucositis, xerostomia, fatigue, nausea and vomiting, with consequent worsening of malnutrition. Nutritional counseling (NC) and oral nutritional supplements (ONS) should be used to increase dietary intake and to prevent therapy-associated weight loss and interruption of radiation therapy. If obstructing cancer and/or mucositis interfere with swallowing, enteral nutrition should be delivered by tube. However, it seems that there is not sufficient evidence to determine the optimal method of enteral feeding. Prophylactic feeding through nasogastric tube or percutaneous gastrostomy to prevent weight loss, reduce dehydration and hospitalizations, and avoid treatment breaks has become relatively common. Compared to reactive feeding (patients are supported with oral nutritional supplements and when it is impossible to maintain nutritional requirements enteral feeding via a NGT or PEG is started), prophylactic feeding does not offer advantages in terms of nutritional outcomes, interruptions of radiotherapy and survival. Overall, it seems that further adequate prospective, randomized studies are needed to define the better nutritional intervention in head and neck cancer patients undergoing chemoradiotherapy.

Keywords: head and neck cancer; chemoradiotherapy; malnutrition; nutrition; nutritional counseling; oral nutritional supplements; enteral nutrition; gastrostomy

1. Introduction

Head and neck cancer (HNC) (cancer of the oral cavity, oropharynx, hypopharynx and larynx) is the seventh most common malignancy in the world [1]. The majority of patients with HNC present with locally advanced disease [1], for which treatment is complex and aggressive, with a therapeutic goal of achieving a cure while minimizing toxicity. The standard of care is multidisciplinary, utilizing bimodality or trimodality therapy where appropriate. Recent advances have led to alterations in radiotherapeutic technologies, the introduction of sequential (induction) systemic chemotherapy, and the inclusion of targeted agents in combination chemotherapy regimens [2].

Head and neck cancer patients are frequently malnourished at the time of diagnosis and prior to the beginning of treatment [3–7]. In addition, chemo-radiotherapy (CRT) causes or exacerbates symptoms, such as alteration or loss of taste, mucositis, xerostomia, fatigue, nausea and vomiting, with consequent worsening of malnutrition [8–12]. It is well known that radiotherapy is invariably associated with mucositis, xerostomia, dysphagia, hematological toxicities and other acute side effects, whose incidence increases when chemotherapy is also administered, and that oral mucositis incidence leads to higher unplanned breaks and delays in radiotherapy administration [13–16]. In addition, in many patients such toxicities may be very severe and even life threatening and may lead to treatment interruptions that are invariably associated with poorer outcome [13–16]. To this regard, it has been shown that during radiotherapy or CRT 55% of the patients may lose an additional 10% or more of body weight [11,12]. Deterioration of the nutritional status results in an increase in CRT-related toxicity and this may increase the prolonged treatment time, which has been associated with poor clinical outcome [17,18].

In the current clinical practice, nutritional counseling with or without oral nutritional supplements patients receiving CRT for head and neck cancer is considered adequate [19] but its real role still remains to be clearly defined with regard to CRT-related toxicity.

If obstructing cancer and/or mucositis interfere with swallowing, enteral nutrition should be delivered by tube. However, it seems that there is not sufficient evidence to determine the optimal method of enteral feeding [19].

Prophylactic feeding through nasogastric tube or percutaneous gastrostomy has become relatively common. It remains to be defined if prophylactic feeding, compared to reactive feeding (patients are supported with oral nutritional supplements and when it is impossible to maintain nutritional requirements enteral feeding via a NGT or PEG is started), offers advantages in terms of nutritional outcomes, interruptions of radiotherapy and survival.

This review aimed to define the role of nutritional counseling, oral nutritional supplements, enteral nutrition through nasogastric tube or gastrostomy, and prophylactic gastrostomy in the prevention and treatment of malnutrition in HNC patients undergoing CRT as well as their impact on CRT-related toxicity and survival.

2. Methods

The following databases were searched for relevant studies up to October 2014: Medline, PubMed, Web of Science, and the Cochrane Library. The search terms and mesh headings included "head and neck neoplasms" OR "head and neck cancer" AND "nutrition" OR "nutrition support" OR "dietary counselling" OR "nutritional counselling" or " nutritional supplements" OR "nutrition therapy" OR "gastrostomy" OR enteral nutrition" OR "enteral feeding" OR "prophylactic gastrostomy" OR "reactive gastrostomy" OR "prophylactic nutrition" OR "prophylactic nutritional support". Reference lists of relevant studies and previous systematic reviews were manually searched for additional articles.

Studies were eligible for inclusion if they were English language papers published in a peer-reviewed journal and met the following inclusion criteria: primary research studies in adult patients (over 18 years of age), included patients with head and neck cancer receiving radiotherapy or radiochemotherapy as the primary treatment, and investigated nutritional interventions in the form of oral supplements or dietary counseling or both or enteral nutrition through nasogastric tube or gastrostomy with primary outcomes, including dietary intake, weight, nutritional status, quality of life, functional status, treatment response, radiotherapy toxicity, or survival. None of the studies with such characteristics was excluded.

3. Nutritional Counseling and Oral Nutritional Supplements

International guidelines suggest that intensive nutritional counseling (NC) and oral nutritional supplements (ONS) should be used to increase dietary intake and to prevent therapy-associated weight loss and interruption of radiation therapy in patients undergoing radiotherapy or chemoradiotherapy of head and neck areas [20–22].

This evidence is based essentially on a randomized study performed in 60 oncology outpatients receiving radiotherapy to the gastrointestinal (12%) or head and neck areas (78%). This study documented statistically smaller deteriorations in weight, nutritional status and global quality of life when intensive, individualized NC and ONS were used instead of standard nutritional care [4,5,21]. Indeed, Ravasco *et al.* [23], two years earlier, randomized 75 HNC patients referred for radiotherapy/chemoradiotherapy to dietary counseling with regular foods (Group 1), usual diet plus supplements (Group 2) and food intake *ad libitum* (Group 3). At three months, Group 1 maintained intakes, whereas Groups 2 and 3 returned to or below baseline levels. In addition, at three months, the reduction of incidence/severity of symptoms (anorexia, nausea/vomiting, xerostomia, and dysgeusia) improved in 90% of the patients in Group 1 *vs.* 67% in Group 2 and 51% in Group 3 ($p < 0.0001$). QOL function scores improved ($p < 0.003$) proportionally with improved nutritional intake and status in Group 1/Group 2 ($p < 0.05$) and worsened in Group 3 ($p < 0.05$).

Thereafter, few studies have been conducted on this topic (Table 1). The recent prospective study of van den Berg *et al.* [24] has clearly confirmed that early and intensive individualized dietary counseling by a dietitian produces clinically relevant effects in terms of decreasing weight loss and malnutrition compared with standard nutritional counseling. All these data are in accordance with previous studies that have evaluated the effects of nutritional counseling and/or ONS in head and neck cancer undergoing radiotherapy only [25,26].

Table 1. Nutritional counseling (NC) and oral nutritional supplements (ONS) in head and neck cancer patients receiving radiotherapy (RT) or chemoradiotherapy (CRT).

Author	Number of Patients	Cancer Therapy	Nutritional Outcome	Interruption of RT
Arnold and Richter, 1989 [25]	Group 1: no nutritional supplements; Group 2: nutritional supplements	RT	No differences between the groups	No differences between the groups
Nayel *et al.*, 1992 [26]	Group 1: 12 pts; radiotherapy alone; Group 2: 11 pts; radiotherapy and ONS	RT	Group 1: in all increase in body weight and in triceps skin-fold thickness, Group 2: 58% had WL ($p = 0.001$)	Group 1: 41.6%; Group 2: 0%; ($p < 0.001$)
Goncalves Diaz *et al.*, 2005 [27]	Group 1: 32 pts; adapted oral diet; Group 2: 16 pts; enteral nutrition via a NG tube (6×/day); Group 3: 16 pts; oral diet associated to ONS between meals (3×/day).	RT	All of the groups presented an increase in the ingestion of calories and proteins ($p < 0.001$).	Not assessed
Ravasco *et al.*, 2005 [23]	Group 1: 25 pts; NC with regular foods; Group 2: 25 pts; usual diet with ONS; Group 3: 25 pts; intake *ad lib.*	CRT	Reduction of anorexia, nausea/vomiting, xerostomia, and dysgeusia: Group 1: 90% of pts; Group 2: 67% of pts; Group 3: 51% of pts	No differences among the groups
Isenring *et al.*, 2007 [21]	Group 1: 31 pts; standard practice; Group 2: 29 pts; individualized NC	CRT	Smaller deteriorations in weight, nutritional status and global quality of life in group 2	Not assessed
Paccagnella *et al.*, 2010 [28]	Group 1: 33 pts; early nutritional intervention before they were submitted to CRT; Group 2: 33 pts; CRT alone	CRT	Group 1: WL (%) 4.4 ± 4.2; Group 2: WL (%) 8.1 ± 4.8; ($p < 0.01$)	Group 1: 30.3%; Group 2: 63.6%; ($p < 0.01$)
Van den Berg, 2010 [24]	Group 1: 20 pts; individual dietary counseling; Group 2: 18 pts; standard dietary counseling	CRT	Group 1: WL (%) 2.3 ± 1.2; Group 2: WL (%) 4.8 ± 2.2	Not assessed
Valentini *et al.*, 2012 [29]	21 pts with NC and ONS	CRT	-	28% for ≥6 days, 28% for 3–5 days and 44% for 0–2 days

In the current clinical practice, NC with or without ONS in patients receiving CRT for head and neck cancer are considered useful but its real role still remains to be clearly defined with regard to CRT-related toxicity. It is possible, in fact, that the improvement of nutritional status obtained through NC and/or ONS may translate in reduced CRT-related toxicity. Unfortunately, data on this issue are few. Among the studies, which included patients receiving radiotherapy, CRT-related toxicity was not assessed in one study and assessed in two (with no differences in one study and with a beneficial effect of ONS on CRT-related toxicity in the other one). Among the studies which included patients receiving chemo-radiotherapy, three did not assess CRT-related toxicity, one found no differences in CRT-related toxicity between patients receiving or not receiving counseling/ONS, and two found such differences. Paccagnella *et al.* [28] showed that the frequency of grade 3–4 mucositis was 45.5% and 39.4% in patients with head and neck cancer undergoing concurrent chemoradiotherapy and receiving, respectively, early nutritional intervention (individualized nutritional counseling and oral supplements or enteral nutrition) or standard practice (general nutrition counseling). However, the percentage of patients who had radiotherapy breaks >5 days for toxicity was significantly lower in the early intervention group than in the standard practice group as well as the number of days of radiotherapy delayed for toxicity and the frequency of hospitalization. The study of Valentini *et al.* [29] has shown that, in patients with head and neck cancer receiving CRT, nutritional counseling combined with ONS was associated with relatively low CRT-related toxicity and with a percentage of patients interrupting anti-neoplastic treatment for 6 or more days lower than 30%.

Taken together, all these data support the concept, suggested by some authors [22,27], that head and neck cancer patients undergoing CRT need early and regular nutritional assessment and interventions during treatment and that dieticians need to adapt to the needs of each patient and provide individualized care. This is particularly true in patients with diabetes, which are not uncommon in such population.

4. Enteral Nutrition via Nasogastric Tube or Gastrostomy

International guidelines also suggest that if an obstructing head and neck cancer interferes with swallowing, enteral nutrition (EN) should be delivered by tube [20]. Tube feeding is also suggested if severe local mucositis is expected, which might interfere with swallowing, e.g., in radio-chemotherapy regimens, including radiation of throat [20].

Tube feeding can either be delivered via the nasogastric tube (NG) or percutaneous gastrostomy (PEG). Because of radiation induced oral and esophageal mucositis, PEG may be preferred and it has been demonstrated clearly that early and appropriate supplementary enteral nutrition via a PEG system is more effective than oral nutrition alone in those cases in which the patient undergoes several weeks of chemotherapy/radiotherapy [30]. However, PEG has a rate of complications that is estimated to be in the range 8%–30%, including local wound infection, occlusion of the tube, leakage from the tube, cellulitis, eczema or hypergranulation tissue [30].

Unfortunately, only three studies have compared NG and PEG in terms of nutritional outcomes, complications, and radiation treatment interruption (Table 2). Of these, two studies were retrospective and one prospective. In the study of Magnè *et al.* [31], 50 HNC patients were managed by PEG and 40 by NG. The feeding methods were found to be equally effective at maintaining body weight and body mass index at time 1 (three weeks) and at time 2 (six weeks). In the study of Mekhail *et al.* [32], NG tubes were placed in 29 patients and PEG in 62. PEG patients had more dysphagia at three months (59% *vs.* 30%, respectively; $p = 0.015$) and at six months (30% *vs.* 8%, respectively; $p = 0.029$) than NG patients. The median tube duration was 28 weeks for PEG patients compared with eight weeks for NG patients, ($p < 0.001$). Twenty-three percent of PEG patients needed pharyngo-esophageal dilatation compared with 4% of NG patients ($p = 0.022$). In the prospective study of Corry *et al.* [33], there were 32 PEG and 73 NGT patients. PEG patients sustained significantly less weight loss at six weeks post-treatment (median 0.8 kg gain *vs.* 3.7 kg loss, $p < 0.001$), but had a high insertion site infection rate (41%), longer median duration of use (146 *vs.* 57 days, $p < 0.001$), and more grade 3 dysphagia in disease-free survivors at six months (25% *vs.* 8%, $p = 0.07$). Patient self-assessed general physical condition and overall quality of life scores were similar in both groups. Overall costs were significantly higher for PEG patients. At six months post-treatment, there was no significant difference between the NGT and PEG groups in complete response at the primary site, weight, dysphagia grade 3 or performance status. Thirty-five percent of evaluable patients in the NGT group (18/52) had ≥10% loss of their body weight compared to 13% (3/23) in the PEG group ($p = 0.09$).

Table 2. Enteral feeding in head and neck cancer patients receiving chemoradiotherapy (CRT): comparison of nasogastric tube (NGT) and percutaneous gastrostomy (PEG). WL, weight loss; QOL, quality of life.

Author	Type of Study	Number of Patients	Cancer Therapy	Nutritional Outcome	Interruption of RT	Other Outcomes
Magnè *et al.*, 2001 [31]	Retrospective	PEG: 50 pts; NGT: 40 pts	CRT	Weight and BMI comparable at week 3 and 6	Not assessed	Better QOL with PEG
Mekhail *et al.*, 2001[32]	Retrospective	PEG: 62 pts; NGT: 29 pts	CRT	Not assessed	Not assessed	Dysphagia more persistent with PEG at 3 and 6 months; By 12 months, difference disappeared
Corry *et al.*, 2009 [33]	Prospective	PEG: 32 pts; NGT: 73 pts	CRT	WL (kg) at 6 weeks: PEG = +0.8 *vs.* NGT = −3.7; $p < 0.001$; WL (kg) at 6 months: PEG = +1 *vs.* NGT = −4.3; $p = 0.04$	Not assessed	PEG patients: high insertion site infection rate (41%), longer duration of use (146 *vs.* 57 days, $p < 0.001$, more grade 3 dysphagia at 6 months; higher costs

Interestingly, long-term swallow function after chemoradiotherapy for head and neck cancer seems to be similar in patients receiving prophylactic gastrostomy and nasogastric tube [34].

Little is known about the number of hospitalizations as well as the costs of the two different feeding approaches. In the study of Corry *et al.* [33], the number of days of hospitalization and costs in the PEG group were significantly higher than in the NGT group. However, if it is considered that PEG is now placed without hospitalization, it is possible that the cost consistently decrease significantly.

It seems that there is not sufficient evidence to determine the optimal method of enteral feeding for patients with head and neck cancer receiving chemoradiotherapy. Further trials comparing the two methods of enteral feeding and including an appropriate number of patients are required.

5. Prophylactic Nutritional Support

In the last decade, the prophylactic feeding (P-FT) through NGT or PEG, before beginning CRT, to prevent weight loss, reduce dehydration and hospitalizations, and avoid treatment breaks has become relatively common. Alternatively, patients are supported with oral nutritional supplements and, when it is impossible to maintain nutritional requirements, enteral feeding via a NGT or PEG is started (reactive feeding; R-FT).

Numerous studies have compared these two approaches as detailed in Table 3. Six studies were retrospective and two prospective, randomized [35–42]. In the majority of these studies, the nutritional outcome was similar in patients receiving prophylactic and reactive feeding. The number of interruptions of anti-cancer treatment was not assessed in two studies and did not differ significantly in five studies. In the study of Lewis *et al.*, patients with P-FT completed a higher proportion of chemotherapy cycles compared to no-FT ($p = 0.002$) and RFT ($p < 0.001$). When assessed, overall and disease-free survival were similar in the different groups of nutritional treatment. One study has shown that quality of life at six months was significantly higher in the group receiving systematic prophylactic gastrostomy [43].

It seems that prophylactic feeding, compared to reactive feeding (patients are supported with oral nutritional supplements and when it is impossible to maintain nutritional requirements enteral feeding via a NGT or PEG is started), does not offer significant advantages in terms of nutritional outcomes, interruptions of radiotherapy and survival. However, considering the limited number of prospective, randomized studies, definitive conclusions cannot be drawn and it is desirable that further investigations will be conducted on this issue in the next future.

Interestingly, Baschnagel *et al.* [44] have recently shown that there was no difference in the PEG tube dependence rates between PEG placed prophylactically *vs.* reactively. However, patients who received a PEG tube reactively had a significantly higher stricture rate and aspiration rate compared to the prophylactic group. In addition, there were significantly fewer hospitalizations in the prophylactic group compared to the reactive group. Overall, when accounting for both PEG placement and hospitalizations, the prophylactic approach was found to be more cost effective.

In 2013, Hughes *et al.* [45] retrospectively examined the data of HNC patients, who underwent CRT for the years before (2005) and after (2007) implementation of internal guidelines, in terms of number of hospitalization and costs. Only five patients (6.5% of all patients treated) in the 2005 cohort received prophylactic gastrostomy tubes compared with 39 patients (44.3%) in the 2007 cohort. Patients in 2007 had significantly fewer hospital admissions, unexpected admissions, and a shorter mean duration of hospital stay in comparison with those in 2005.

Noteworthy, a recent retrospective study has identified independent risk factors (BMI >25, a tumor classification ≥ 3, a cumulative cisplatin dose of 200 mg/m^2) associated with symptomatic requirement for the reactive placement of a PEG tube [46].

Table 3. Prophylactic feeding in head and neck cancer patients receiving chemoradiotherapy (CRT). P-PEG, prophylactic percutaneous gastrostomy; R-PEG, reactive percutaneous gastrostomy. No-FT, no feeding tube; NGT, nasogastric tube; NC, nutritional counselling; ONS, oral nutritional supplements.

Author	Type of Study	Cancer Therapy	Number of Patients	Nutritional Treatment	Nutritional Outcome	Interruption of RT	Survival
Salas et al., 2009 [43]	Randomized trial	CRT	39	P-PEG: 21 pts; R-PEG: 18 pts	Similar decrease of BMI at 6 months in the two groups	Not assessed	Survival not assessed. Better QOL at 6 months in the P-PEG group
Nugent et al., 2010 [41]	Retrospective	CRT	76	ONS: 26 pts; NGT: 18 pts; P-PEG: 21 pts; R-PEG: 11 pts	WL% at end of treatment:ONS: 6.1NG-tube: 8.5 P-PEG: 4.6; T-PEG:8.7; (p = NS)	No differences between the groups	Not assessed
Chen et al., 2010 [42]	Retrospective	CRT	120	Control: 20 pts; P-PEG: 70 pts	WL% at end of treatment: Control: 14; P-PEG: 8 ($p <$ 0.001); WL% at 3 months: Control: 8P-PEG: 5; (p = 0.34)	No differences between the groups (p = 0.54)	No significant differences in the 3-year overall and disease-free survival
Silander et al., 2012 [40]	Randomized trial	CRT	134	NC (+NGT): 70 pts; P-PEG: 64 pts	Same proportion of patients who had a 10 % weight loss at 3, 6 and 12 months	No differences between the groups (p = 0.08)	No differences in 2-year survival between the groups (p = 0.40)
Williams et al., 2012 [39]	Retrospective	CRT	104	NGT: 21 pts; P-PEG: 71 pts; R-PEG: 12 pts	No differences in weight loss at the end of treatment and at 6 months post-radiotherapy (p = 0.23).	No differences between the groups (p = 0.47).	No significant differences in disease free and overall survival between the groups (p = 0.90 and p = 0.13, respectively)
Olson et al., 2013 [38]	Retrospective	CRT	445	Center A, prefers R-PEG; Center B, prefers P-PEG;	Same % of patients with 10% weight loss at 1 year in the two centers	Not assessed	No significant differences in the overall survival
Lewis et al., 2013 [37]	Retrospective	CRT	109	Control: 50 pts; P-PEG:25 pts; R-PEG: 34 pts	Weight loss (%): Control: 15.2; P-PEG: 2.4; R-PEG: 10.4	Patients with P- PEG completed a higher proportion of chemotherapy cycles compared to control (p = 0.002) and R- PEG (p <0.001).	Not assessed
Kramer et al., 2014 [36]	Retrospective	CRT	74	P-PEG: 56 pts; R-PEG: 300 pts	No difference in weight loss (%) at 2, 6, 12 months.	Not assessed.	No difference in survival or disease control

31

6. Conclusions

Head and neck cancer patients undergoing chemoradiotherapy are at risk of malnutrition before and during treatment. Nutritional counseling and oral nutritional supplements should be used to increase dietary intake and to prevent therapy-associated weight loss and interruption of radiation therapy. If obstructing cancer and/or mucositis interfere with swallowing, enteral nutrition should be delivered by tube. However, it seems that there is not sufficient evidence to determine the optimal method of enteral feeding. Prophylactic feeding through nasogastric tube or percutaneous gastrostomy to prevent weight loss, reduce dehydration and hospitalizations, and avoid treatment breaks has become relatively common. However, compared to reactive feeding (patients are supported with oral nutritional supplements and when it is impossible to maintain nutritional requirements enteral feeding via a NGT or PEG is started), prophylactic feeding does not offer advantages in terms of nutritional outcomes, interruptions of radiotherapy and survival.

Overall, it seems that further adequate prospective, randomized studies are needed to define the better nutritional intervention in head and neck cancer patients undergoing chemoradiotherapy and to eventually change the current practice, having in mind that the nutritional treatment of these patients is complex and requires a multidisciplinary approach.

Conflicts of Interest: The author declare no conflict of interest.

References

1. World Health Organization. *World Cancer Report 2014 (ePUB)*; World Health Organization Press: Lyon, France, 2014.
2. Denaro, N.; Russi, E.G.; Adamo, V.; Merlano, M.C. State-of-the-art and emerging treatment options in the management of head and neck cancer, news from 2013. *Oncology* **2014**, *86*, 212–229. [PubMed]
3. De Luis, D.A.; Izaola, O.; Aller, R. Nutritional status in head and neck cancer patients. *Eur. Rev. Med. Pharmacol. Sci.* **2007**, *11*, 239–243.
4. Isenring, E.A.; Capra, S.; Bauer, J.D. Nutrition intervention is beneficial in oncology outpatients receiving radiotherapy to the gastrointestinal or head and neck area. *Br. J. Cancer* **2004**, *91*, 447–452. [CrossRef] [PubMed]
5. Isenring, E.; Capra, S.; Bauer, J. Patient satisfaction is rated higher by radiation oncology outpatients receiving nutrition intervention compared with usual care. *J. Hum. Nutr. Diet.* **2004**, *17*, 145–152. [CrossRef] [PubMed]
6. Van Wayenburg, C.A.; Rasmussen-Conrad, E.L.; van den Berg, M.G.; Merkx, M.A.; van Staveren, W.A.; van Weel, C.; van Binsbergen, J.J. Weight loss in head and neck cancer patients little noticed in general practice. *J. Prim. Health Care* **2010**, *2*, 16–21.
7. Van Leeuwen, P.A.; Kuik, D.J.; Klop, W.M.; Sauerwein, H.P.; Snow, G.B.; Quak, J.J. The impact of nutritional status on the prognoses of patients with advanced head and neck cancer. *Cancer* **1999**, *86*, 519–527.
8. Bonner, J.A.; Harari, P.M.; Giralt, J.; Azarnia, N.; Shin, D.M.; Cohen, R.B.; Jones, C.U.; Sur, R.; Raben, D.; Jassem, J.; *et al.* Radiotherapy plus cetuximab for squamous-cell carcinoma of the head and neck. *N. Engl. J. Med.* **2006**, *354*, 567–578. [CrossRef] [PubMed]
9. Brizel, D.M.; Albers, M.E.; Fisher, S.R.; Scher, R.L.; Richtsmeier, W.J.; Hars, V.; George, S.L.; Huang, A.T.; Prosnitz, L.R. Hyperfractionated irradiation with or without concurrent chemotherapy for locally advanced head and neck cancer. *N. Engl. J. Med.* **1998**, *18*, 1798–1804. [CrossRef]
10. Colasanto, J.M.; Prasad, P.; Nash, M.A.; Decker, R.H.; Wilson, L.D. Nutritional support of patients undergoing radiation therapy for head and neck cancer. *Oncology* **2005**, *19*, 371–379. [PubMed]
11. Ng, K.; Leung, S.F.; Johnson, P.J.; Woo, J. Nutritional consequences of radiotherapy in nasopharynx cancer patients. *Nutr. Cancer* **2004**, *49*, 156–161. [CrossRef] [PubMed]
12. Silver, H.J.; Dietrich, M.S.; Murphy, B.A. Changes in body mass, energy balance, physical function, and inflammatory state in patients with locally advanced head and neck cancer treated with concurrent chemoradiation after low-dose induction chemotherapy. *Head Neck* **2007**, *29*, 893–900. [CrossRef] [PubMed]

13. Bernier, J.; Domenge, C.; Ozsahin, M.; Matuszewska, K.; Lefèbvre, J.L.; Greiner, R.H.; Giralt, J.; Maingon, P.; Rolland, F.; Bolla, M.; *et al.* Postoperative irradiation with or without concomitant chemotherapy for locally advanced head and neck cancer. *N. Engl. J. Med.* **2004**, *350*, 1945–1952. [CrossRef] [PubMed]

14. Bieri, S.; Bentzen, S.M.; Huguenin, P.; Allal, A.S.; Cozzi, L.; Landmann, C.; Monney, M.; Bernier, J. Early morbidity after radiotherapy with or without chemotherapy in advanced head and neck cancer. Experience from four nonrandomized studies. *Strahlenther. Onkol.* **2003**, *179*, 390–395. [PubMed]

15. Cooper, J.S.; Pajak, T.F.; Forastiere, A.A.; Jacobs, J.; Campbell, B.H.; Saxman, S.B.; Kish, J.A.; Kim, H.E.; Cmelak, A.J.; Rotman, M.; *et al.* Long-term follow-up of the RTOG 9501/intergroup phase III trial, postoperative concurrent radiation therapy and chemotherapy in high-risk squamous cell carcinoma of the head and neck. *Int. J. Radiat. Oncol. Biol. Phys.* **2012**, *84*, 1198–1205. [CrossRef] [PubMed]

16. Lin, A.; Jabbari, S.; Worden, F.P.; Bradford, C.R.; Chepeha, D.B.; Teknos, T.N.; Liao, J.J.; Nyquist, G.G.; Tsien, C.; Schipper, M.J.; *et al.* Metabolic abnormalities associated with weight loss during chemoirradiation of head-and-neck cancer. *Int. J. Radiat. Oncol. Biol. Phys.* **2005**, *63*, 1413–1418. [CrossRef] [PubMed]

17. Rosenthal, D.I. Consequences of mucositis-induced treatment breaks and dose reductions on head and neck cancer treatment outcomes. *J. Support. Oncol.* **2007**, *9* (Suppl. 4), 23–31.

18. Vera-Llonch, M.; Oster, G.; Hagiwara, M.; Sonis, S. Oral mucositis in patients undergoing radiation treatment for head and neck carcinoma. *Cancer* **2006**, *106*, 329–336. [CrossRef] [PubMed]

19. Garg, S.; Yoo, J.; Winquist, E. Nutritional support for head and neck cancer patients receiving radiotherapy: A systematic review. *Support. Care Cancer* **2010**, *8*, 667–677. [CrossRef]

20. Arends, J.; Bodoky, G.; Bozzetti, F.; Fearon, K.; van Bokhorst-de van der Schueren, M.A.; Muscaritoli, M.; Selga, G.; von Meyenfeldt, M.; DGEM (German Society for Nutritional Medicine); Zürcher, G.; *et al.* ESPEN Guidelines on Enteral Nutrition, Non-surgical oncology. *Clin. Nutr.* **2006**, *25*, 245–259. [CrossRef] [PubMed]

21. Isenring, E.A.; Bauer, J.D.; Capra, S. Nutrition support using the American Dietetic Association medical nutrition therapy protocol for radiation oncology patients improves dietary intake compared with standard practice. *J. Am. Diet. Assoc.* **2007**, *107*, 404–412. [CrossRef] [PubMed]

22. Bauer, D.J.; Ash, S.; Davidson, L.W.; Hill, M.J.; Brown, T.; Isenring, A.E.; Reeves, M. Evidence based practice guidelines for the nutritional management of patients receiving radiation therapy of the Dietitians Association of Australia. *Nutr. Diet.* **2008**, *65*, 1–20.

23. Ravasco, P.; Monteiro-Grillo, I.; Marques Vidal, P.; Camilo, M.E. Impact of nutrition on outcome, a prospective randomized controlled trial in patients with head and neck cancer undergoing radiotherapy. *Head Neck* **2005**, *27*, 659–668. [CrossRef] [PubMed]

24. Van den Berg, M.G.; Rasmussen-Conrad, E.L.; Wei, K.H.; Lintz-Luidens, H.; Kaanders, J.H.; Merkx, M.A. Comparison of the effect of individual dietary counselling and of standard nutritional care on weight loss in patients with head and neck cancer undergoing radiotherapy. *Br. J. Nutr.* **2010**, *104*, 872–877. [CrossRef] [PubMed]

25. Arnold, C.; Richter, M.P. The effect of oral nutritional supplements on head and neck cancer. *Int. J. Radiat. Oncol. Biol. Phys.* **1989**, *16*, 1595–1599. [CrossRef] [PubMed]

26. Nayel, H.; el-Ghoneimy, E.; el-Haddad, S. Impact of nutritional supplementation on treatment delay and morbidity inpatients with head and neck tumors treated with irradiation. *Nutrition* **1992**, *8*, 13–18. [PubMed]

27. Gonçalves Dias, M.C.; de Fátima Nunes Marucci, M.; Nadalin, W.; Waitzberg, D.L. Nutritional intervention improves the caloric and proteic ingestion of head and neck cancer patients under radiotherapy. *Nutr. Hosp.* **2005**, *20*, 320–325. [PubMed]

28. Paccagnella, A.; Morello, M.; da Mosto, M.C.; Baruffi, C.; Marcon, M.L.; Gava, A.; Baggio, V.; Lamon, S.; Babare, R.; Rosti, G.; *et al.* Early nutritional intervention improves treatment tolerance and outcomes in head and neck cancer patients undergoing concurrent chemoradiotherapy. *Support. Care Cancer* **2010**, *18*, 837–845. [CrossRef] [PubMed]

29. Valentini, V.; Marazzi, F.; Bossola, M.; Miccichè, F.; Nardone, L.; Balducci, M.; Dinapoli, N.; Bonomo, P.; Autorino, R.; Silipigni, S.; *et al.* Nutritional counselling and oral nutritional supplements in head and neck cancer patients undergoing chemoradiotherapy. *J. Hum. Nutr. Diet.* **2012**, *25*, 201–208. [CrossRef] [PubMed]

30. Löser, C.; Aschl, G.; Hébuterne, X.; Mathus-Vliegen, E.M.; Muscaritoli, M.; Niv, Y.; Rollins, H.; Singer, P.; Skelly, R.H. ESPEN guidelines on artificial enteral nutrition—Percutaneous endoscopic gastrostomy (PEG). *Clin. Nutr.* **2005**, *24*, 848–861. [CrossRef] [PubMed]

31. Magné, N.; Marcy, P.Y.; Foa, C.; Falewee, M.N.; Schneider, M.; Demard, F.; Bensadoun, R.J. Comparison between nasogastric tube feeding and percutaneous fluoroscopic gastrostomy in advanced head and neck cancer patients. *Eur. Arch. Otorhinolaryngol.* **2001**, *258*, 89–92. [CrossRef] [PubMed]

32. Mekhail, T.M.; Adelstein, D.J.; Rybicki, L.A.; Larto, M.A.; Saxton, J.P.; Lavertu, P. Enteral nutrition during the treatment of head and neck carcinoma: Is a percutaneous endoscopic gastrostomy tube preferable to a nasogastric tube? *Cancer* **2001**, *91*, 1785–1790. [CrossRef] [PubMed]

33. Corry, J.; Poon, W.; McPhee, N.; Milner, A.D.; Cruickshank, D.; Porceddu, S.V.; Rischin, D.; Peters, L.J. Prospective study of percutaneous endoscopic gastrostomy tubes *vs.* nasogastric tubes for enteral feeding in patients with head and neck cancer undergoing (chemo)radiation. *Head Neck* **2009**, *31*, 867–876. [CrossRef] [PubMed]

34. Prestwich, R.J.; Teo, M.T.; Gilbert, A.; Williams, G.; Dyker, K.E.; Sen, M. Long-term swallow function after chemoradiotherapy for oropharyngeal cancer: The influence of a prophylactic gastrostomy or reactive nasogastric tube. *Clin. Oncol. (R. CollRadiol.)* **2014**, *26*, 103–109. [CrossRef]

35. Lee, J.H.; Machtay, M.; Unger, L.D.; Weinstein, G.S.; Weber, R.S.; Chalian, A.A.; Rosenthal, D.I. (1998) Prophylactic gastrostomy tubes in patients undergoing intensive radiation irradiation for cancer of the head and neck. *Arch. Otolaryngol. Head Neck Surg.* **1998**, *124*, 871–875. [CrossRef] [PubMed]

36. Kramer, S.; Newcomb, M.; Hessler, J.; Siddiqui, F. Prophylactic *vs.* reactive PEG tube placement in head and neck cancer. *Otolaryngol. Head Neck Surg.* **2014**, *150*, 407–412. [CrossRef] [PubMed]

37. Lewis, S.L.; Brody, R.; Touger-Decker, R.; Parrott, J.S.; Epstein, J. Feeding tube use in head and neck cancer patients. *Head Neck* **2013**. [CrossRef]

38. Olson, R.; Karam, I.; Wilson, G.; Bowman, A.; Lee, C.; Wong, F. Population-based comparison of two feeding tube approaches for head and neck cancer patients receiving concurrent systemic-radiation therapy: Is a prophylactic feeding tube approach harmful or helpful? *Support. Care Cancer.* **2013**, *21*, 3433–3439. [CrossRef] [PubMed]

39. Williams, G.F.; Teo, M.T.; Sen, M.; Dyker, K.E.; Coyle, C.; Prestwich, R.J. Enteral feeding outcomes after chemoradiotherapy for oropharynx cancer: A role for a prophylactic gastrostomy? *Oral Oncol.* **2012**, *48*, 434–440. [CrossRef] [PubMed]

40. Silander, E.; Nyman, J.; Bove, M.; Johansson, L.; Larsson, S.; Hammerlid, E. Impact of prophylactic percutaneous endoscopic gastrostomy on malnutrition and quality of life in patients with head and neck cancer: A randomized study. *Head Neck* **2012**, *34*, 1–9. [CrossRef] [PubMed]

41. Nugent, B.; Parker, M.J.; McIntyre, I.A. Nasogastric tube feeding and percutaneous endoscopic gastrostomy tube feeding in patients with head and neck cancer. *J. Hum. Nutr. Diet.* **2010**, *23*, 277–284. [CrossRef] [PubMed]

42. Chen, A.M.; Li, B.Q.; Lau, D.H.; Farwell, D.G.; Luu, Q.; Stuart, K.; Newman, K.; Purdy, J.A.; Vijayakumar, S. Evaluating the role of prophylactic gastrostomy tube placement prior to definitive chemoradiotherapy for head and neck cancer. *Int. J. Radiat. Oncol. Biol. Phys.* **2010**, *78*, 1026–1032. [CrossRef] [PubMed]

43. Salas, S.; Baumstarck-Barrau, K.; Alfonsi, M.; Digue, L.; Bagarry, D.; Feham, N.; Bensadoun, R.J.; Pignon, T.; Loundon, A.; Deville, J.L.; *et al.* Impact of the prophylactic gastrostomy for unresectable squamous cell head and neck carcinomas treated with radio-chemotherapy on quality of life: Prospective randomized trial. *Radiother. Oncol.* **2009**, *93*, 503–509. [CrossRef] [PubMed]

44. Baschnagel, A.M.; Yadav, S.; Marina, O.; Parzuchowski, A.; Lanni, T.B., Jr.; Warner, J.N.; Parzuchowski, J.S.; Ignatius, R.T.; Akervall, J.; Chen, P.Y.; *et al.* Toxicities and costs of placing prophylactic and reactive percutaneous gastrostomy tubes in patients with locally advanced head and neck cancers treated with chemoradiotherapy. *Head Neck* **2014**, *36*, 1155–1161. [CrossRef] [PubMed]

45. Hughes, B.G.; Jain, V.K.; Brown, T.; Spurgin, A.L.; Hartnett, G.; Keller, J.; Tripcony, L.; Appleyard, M.; Hodge, R. Decreased hospital stay and significant cost savings after routine use of prophylactic gastrostomy for high-risk patients with head and neck cancer receiving chemoradiotherapy at a tertiary cancer institution. *Head Neck* **2013**, *35*, 436–442. [CrossRef] [PubMed]

46. Strom, T.; Trotti, A.M.; Kish, J.; Rao, N.G.; McCaffrey, J.; Padhya, T.A.; Lin, H.Y.; Fulp, W.; Caudell, J.J. Risk factors for percutaneous endoscopic gastrostomy tube placement during chemoradiotherapy for oropharyngeal cancer. *JAMA Otolaryngol. Head Neck Surg.* **2013**, *139*, 1242–1246. [CrossRef] [PubMed]

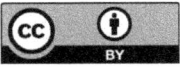

nutrients

MDPI

Review

Guidelines for Feeding Very Low Birth Weight Infants

Sourabh Dutta *, Balpreet Singh, Lorraine Chessell, Jennifer Wilson, Marianne Janes, Kimberley McDonald, Shaneela Shahid, Victoria A. Gardner, Aune Hjartarson, Margaret Purcha, Jennifer Watson, Chris de Boer, Barbara Gaal and Christoph Fusch

Division of Neonatology, Department of Pediatrics, McMaster University Children's Hospital, Hamilton L8S4L8, Ontario, Canada; drbalpreetsingh@yahoo.com (B.S.); chessell@HHSC.CA (L.C.); wilsonj@HHSC.CA (J.W.); janes@HHSC.CA (M.J.); mcdonk@HHSC.CA (K.M.); shahidsattar75@yahoo.com (S.S.); gardner@hhsc.ca (V.A.G.); hjartar@hhsc.ca (A.H.); purcham@HHSC.CA (M.P.); watsonje@hhsc.ca (J.W.); deboerc@hhsc.ca (C.B.); B.Gaal@bell.net (B.G.); fusch@mcmaster.ca (C.F.)

* Author to whom correspondence should be addressed; sdutta@mcmaster.ca; Tel.: +1-905-521-2100; Fax: 1-905-521-5007.

Received: 16 November 2014; Accepted: 19 December 2014; Published: 8 January 2015

Abstract: Despite the fact that feeding a very low birth weight (VLBW) neonate is a fundamental and inevitable part of its management, this is a field which is beset with controversies. Optimal nutrition improves growth and neurological outcomes, and reduces the incidence of sepsis and possibly even retinopathy of prematurity. There is a great deal of heterogeneity of practice among neonatologists and pediatricians regarding feeding VLBW infants. A working group on feeding guidelines for VLBW infants was constituted in McMaster University, Canada. The group listed a number of important questions that had to be answered with respect to feeding VLBW infants, systematically reviewed the literature, critically appraised the level of evidence, and generated a comprehensive set of guidelines. These guidelines form the basis of this state-of-art review. The review touches upon trophic feeding, nutritional feeding, fortification, feeding in special circumstances, assessment of feed tolerance, and management of gastric residuals, gastro-esophageal reflux, and glycerin enemas.

Keywords: feeding; very low birth weight; neonate; review

1. Introduction

Adequate nutrition is essential for the optimal growth and health of very low birth weight (VLBW) infants. Enteral nutrition is preferred to total parenteral nutrition (TPN) because the former avoids complications related to vascular catheterization, sepsis, adverse effects of TPN, and fasting. Early parenteral nutrition in these babies remains critical and should be used as an adjunct to enteral nutrition. The overarching goal while feeding VLBW infants (VLBWI) is to reach full enteral feeding in the shortest time, while maintaining optimal growth and nutrition and avoiding the adverse consequences of rapid advancement of feeding. Attaining this goal is more difficult than it sounds, and controversies abound.

A multi-disciplinary working group in McMaster University (comprised of staff neonatologists, fellows, nutritionists, nurse practitioners, nurses, lactation consultants, and occupational therapists) conducted a structured literature search, critically appraised the evidence, presented it to a wider group of neonatologists, and came up with practical suggestions to feed VLBWI—the basis for this review. There are some areas where there is limited evidence, and in these areas we have suggested reasonable approaches based on expert consensus. Wherever possible, we have stated the level of evidence (LOE) as per the Centre for Evidence-based Medicine, United Kingdom [1]. The outline of the LOE for therapy trials is as follows:

1a   Systematic review (with homogeneity) of randomized controlled trials (RCT)

1b   Individual RCT with narrow confidence interval (CI)

2a   Systematic review (with homogeneity) of cohort studies

2b   Individual cohort studies and low-quality RCTs

3a   Systematic review (with homogeneity) of case-control studies

3b   Individual case-control studies

4   Case series, poor-quality cohort and poor-quality case-control studies

5   Expert opinion without explicit critical appraisal

If a minus sign is suffixed (e.g., 1a− or 1b−), it denotes either a single study with wide CI or a systematic review with troublesome heterogeneity.

2. Time to Reach Full Feeds

2.1. Suggestion

Aim to reach full enteral feeding (~150–180 mL/kg/day) by about two weeks in babies weighing <1000 g at birth and by about one week in babies weighing 1000–1500 g by implementing evidence-based feeding protocols. It may be noted that some babies, especially those less than 1000 grams, will not tolerate larger volumes of feedings (such as 180 mL/kg/day or more) and thus may need individualization.

2.2. Rationale

Reaching full enteral feeding faster results in earlier removal of vascular catheters, and less sepsis and other catheter-related complications (LOE 2b) [2–4]. Standardized feeding protocols improve outcomes in VLBWI [4,5]. Reaching full feeds within a week is achievable—in an RCT on VLBWI, the median time to reach 170 mL/kg/day was 7 days after fast advancement of enteral feeding, with no increase in apneas, feed interruptions, and intolerance [6].

3. Frequency of Feeds

3.1. Suggestion

Administer three-hourly feeds for babies weighing >1250 g. There is not enough evidence to choose between two-hourly *versus* three-hourly feeds for babies weighing ≤1250 g.

3.2. Rationale

In an RCT, 92 neonates weighing <1750 g were allocated to either three- or two-hourly feeds [7]. The incidence of feed intolerance, apnea, hypoglycemia, and necrotizing enterocolitis (NEC) did not significantly differ, and nursing time spent on feeding was significantly less in the three-hourly group (LOE 2b).

Two retrospective studies on this issue were contradictory. In one that compared 2-h and 3-h enteral feeding in ELBW babies, the time to full enteral feeding, enteral morbidity, hospital stay, and growth parameters were similar in the two groups (LOE 4) [8]. In another, VLBWI (mean birth weight ~1200 g) fed twice hourly reached full feeds faster, received less prolonged TPN, and were less likely to have feeds held, compared to those fed three times hourly (LOE 4) [9]. Putting this limited information together, we propose that babies weighing ≥1250 g be fed three times hourly and those weighing <1250 g preferably twice hourly.

4. Trophic Feeds: Time of Starting, Volume, Duration

4.1. Suggestion

Trophic feeds are defined as minimal volumes of milk feeds (10–15 mL/kg/day). Start trophic feeds preferably within 24 h of life. Exercise caution in extremely preterm, extremely low birth weight (ELBW), or growth-restricted infants. If, by 24–48 h, no maternal or donor milk is available, consider formula milk. There is not enough evidence to recommend the maximum duration of trophic feeding before starting nutritional feeds.

4.2. Rationale

In a systematic review (nine trials, 754 VLBWI), the actual volume of trophic feeds ranged from 10 to 25 mL/kg/day; and onset from day one of life onwards [10]. Early introduction of trophic feeds compared to fasting had a non-significant trend towards reaching full feeds earlier (mean difference − 1.05 days (95% CI −2.61, 0.51)) and no difference in NEC (LOE 1a−). More data is required before one can generalize these findings to extremely preterm, ELBW, or growth-restricted infants.

There was no subgroup analysis on formula milk. Among the included studies, there were two studies in which trophic feeding was provided exclusively by preterm formula (LOE 1b−) [11,12]. In both, the trophic feeding group had less feeding intolerance and reached full feeds faster without increase in NEC. Hence, formula milk may be used after exhausting other options. We suggest a reasonable waiting period of 24–48 h for obtaining maternal or donor milk.

In a systematic review (seven trials, 964 VLBWI) on timing of introduction of nutritional enteral feeding to prevent NEC, early introduction of progressive enteral feeding (1 to 2 days of age) did not increase the risk of NEC (typical relative risk (RR) 0.92 (95% CI 0.64, 1.34)), mortality (typical RR 1.26 (95% CI 0.78, 2.01)), or feed intolerance (LOE 1a) [13]. We converted this into a practical suggestion of the maximum number of days for trophic feeding before introducing progressive enteral feeding.

5. Contraindications for Trophic Feeds

5.1. Suggestion

Withhold trophic feeds in intestinal obstruction or a setting for intestinal obstruction or ileus.

Asphyxia, respiratory distress, sepsis, hypotension, glucose disturbances, ventilation, and umbilical lines are not contraindications for trophic feeds.

5.2. Rationale

The studies included in a Cochrane review included VLBWI with asphyxia, respiratory distress, sepsis, hypotension, glucose disturbances, ventilation, and umbilical lines, without any excess adverse effects being reported (LOE 1a−) [10].

6. Nutritional Feeds: Day of Starting, Volume, Frequency, Increase

6.1. Suggestion

In babies weighing <1 kg at birth, start nutritional feeds at 15–20 mL/kg/day and increase by 15–20 mL/kg/day. If the feeds are tolerated for around 2–3 days, consider increasing faster. For babies weighing ≥1 kg at birth, start nutritional feeds at 30 mL/kg/day and increase by 30 mL/kg/day.

6.2. Rationale

A Cochrane review (four RCTs, 588 subjects) compared slow daily increments (ranging from 15 to 20 mL/kg/day) *versus* fast daily increments of enteral feeding volume (ranging from 30 to 35 mL/kg/day) (LOE 1a) [14]. Fast increment did not increase the risk of NEC (pooled RR 0.97 (95% CI 0.54, 1.74)), mortality (pooled RR 1.41 (95% CI 0.81, 2.74)), or interruption of feeds (pooled RR 1.29 (95% CI 0.90, 1.85)). The trials individually reported that the fast daily increment group regained birth weight and reached full feeds faster (LOE 1b and 2b). As there was no subgroup analysis of ELBW babies, we suggest starting with a lower feed volume in ELBW babies—as in the control arm (15–20 mL/kg/day)—until more studies are available.

7. Type of Milk for Starting Feeds

7.1. Suggestion

The first choice is own mother's expressed breast milk or colostrum. This should preferably be fresh; if not, provide previously frozen milk in the same sequence in which it was expressed.
Second choice: donor human milk.
Third choice: preterm formula.

7.2. Rationale

Freshly expressed human milk has numerous benefits for preterm babies [15]. Although there is no direct evidence comparing fresh *versus* frozen mother's milk, the use of fresh milk makes sense because of the depletion of commensals, immune cells, immune factors, and enzyme activity that occurs with freezing. Neonates who receive an exclusively human milk-based diet (mother's milk or donor human milk with human milk-based fortifier) have significantly lower rates of NEC compared to those who receive preterm formula or human milk with a bovine milk-based fortifier (LOE 1b) [16]. In another RCT, preterm infants who received an exclusively human milk diet (donor human milk and human milk-based human milk fortifier) had a lower incidence of NEC (21% *versus* 3%, $p = 0.08$) and surgical NEC ($p = 0.04$) compared to infants who received bovine milk-based preterm formula [17]. The use of donor human milk (while continuing bovine milk-based fortifier) *versus* preterm formula as a substitute for mother's own milk does not reduce the rates of NEC [18]. The prohibitively high cost of human milk-based human milk fortifier is often quoted as an obstacle to using an exclusively human milk diet; however, a cost-effectiveness analysis showed that use of exclusively human milk-based products resulted in shorter duration of hospitalization (less by an average of 3.9 days in neonatal intensive care unit (NICU)) and savings of $8167 per extremely premature infant ($p < 0.0001$) because of the reduction in NEC [19].

8. Feeding Small for Gestational Age (SGA) Babies with/without History of Absent/Reversed End Diastolic Umbilical Flow (AREDF)

8.1. Suggestion

If the abdominal examination is normal, start feeding within 24 h of life, but advance slowly with volumes at the lowest end of the range. Advance feeds extremely slowly in the first 10 days among preterm SGA babies with gestation <29 weeks and AREDF. Make every effort to feed human milk, especially in SGA babies with AREDF and gestation <29 weeks.

8.2. Rationale

Mihatsch *et al.* [20] fed 124 VLBWI (35 had intra-uterine growth retardation (IUGR)) with a standardized protocol (LOE 2b). There was no statistical difference in the age to reach full feeds in the IUGR and non-IUGR groups ($p = 0.6$). In a multiple regression model, increased umbilical artery resistance, brain sparing, Apgar scores, umbilical artery pH, and IUGR did not predict the age to reach full feeds. In an RCT on SGA preterm babies (gestation of 27–34 weeks) who had abnormal antenatal umbilical Doppler flows, the incidence of NEC and feeding intolerance was not significantly different ($p = 0.35$ and $p = 0.53$, respectively) between the early feeders ($n = 42$; median age 2 days) and delayed feeders ($n = 42$; 7 days) (LOE 2b) [21].

In an RCT on preterm SGA infants, comparing minimal enteral feeding and no enteral feeding for five days, there was no difference in the rate of NEC ($p = 0.76$) and there was a trend towards shorter NICU stay in the enteral feeding group ($p = 0.2$) (LOE 2b) [22].

In the Abnormal Doppler Enteral Prescription Trial (ADEPT) RCT, 402 preterm SGA infants (<35 weeks gestation, birth weight < 10th centile) with absent or reversed end diastolic umbilical blood flow and cerebral redistribution were allocated to early or late onset of enteral feeding (Day 2 or 6, respectively) (LOE 1b) [23].The early feeding group reached full enteral feeds faster than the late feeding group (median (IQR) days: 18 (15–24) *versus* 21 (19–27), respectively; $p = 0.003$). There was no difference in the incidence of all-stage NEC (18% *versus* 15%, respectively; $p = 0.42$) and stage II–III NEC. Infants in the early feeding group had a significantly shorter duration of total parenteral nutrition (median difference 3 days, $p < 0.001$), a shorter duration of high dependency care ($p = 0.002$), and a lower incidence of cholestasis ($p = 0.02$). Eighty-six (21%) infants in this trial were below 29 weeks of gestation. The statistical test of interaction between treatment group and gestational age group (<29 weeks *versus* ≥29 weeks) was non-significant for age to reach full feeds ($p = 0.38$) and incidence of all stage NEC ($p = 0.47$), suggesting that the treatment effect was consistent across subgroups. The investigators published additional analysis from the ADEPT trial comparing infants of <29 weeks and ≥29 weeks of gestation [24]. The former group took significantly longer to reach full feeds compared to the latter (median age 28 days (Inter-quartile range (IQR) 22–40) *versus* 19 days (IQR 17–23), respectively; hazard ratio 0.35 (95% CI 0.3, 0.5)) and had a significantly higher incidence of NEC (39% *versus* 10%, respectively; RR 3.7 (95% CI 2.4, 5.7)). Infants <29 weeks in this trial tolerated very little milk in the first 10 days. Exclusive human milk feeding was the only protective factor.

9. Feeding Babies on Non-Invasive Ventilation

9.1. Suggestion

Increase feeds cautiously. Do not rely on abdominal distension as a sign of feeding intolerance, especially in babies weighing <1000 g.

9.2. Rationale

Non-invasive ventilation can cause abdominal distension, and nasal continuous positive airway pressure (nCPAP) decreases pre-and post-prandial intestinal blood flow in preterm infants (LOE 4) [25]. Jaile *et al.* [26] compared 25 premature infants on nCPAP with 29 premature infants not on CPAP (LOE 2b). Gaseous bowel distension due to CPAP developed in 83% of infants below 1000 g *versus* 14% of those weighing ≥1000 g. No cases of NEC were reported in the study; however, the sample size was too small to draw conclusions about NEC.

10. Feeding Babies with Systemic Arterial Hypotension

10.1. Suggestion

There is not enough evidence to make a suggestion.

10.2. Rationale

There is no published literature on feeding policies during systemic arterial hypotension.

11. Feeding Babies on Indomethacin or Ibuprofen

11.1. Suggestion

If the neonate is already on minimal feeds, continue to give trophic feeds until the indomethacin course finishes. If the neonate is fasting, introduce trophic feeds with human milk as per Section 3.

While there are no RCTs comparing feeding during indomethacin therapy *versus* ibuprofen, indirect evidence suggests ibuprofen may be the safer of the two.

11.2. Rationale

In the Ductus Arteriosus Feed or Fast with Indomethacin or Ibuprofen (DAFFII) trial, 117 infants (26.3 ± 1.9 weeks) who were on ≤ 60 mL/kg/day feeds and required treatment for patent ductus arteriosus (PDA) (75% to 80% received indomethacin) were randomized at 6.5 ± 3.9 days to receive trophic feeds or no feeds during the drug administration period [27]. Infants randomized to the trophic feeding subsequently required fewer days to reach 120 mL/kg/day (10.3 ± 6.6 days *vs.* 13.1 ± 7.8 days, $p < 0.05$). There is one retrospective study on 64 preterm infants (<29 weeks of gestation), half of whom had received indomethacin for PDA (LOE 4) [28]. There were no differences between the groups regarding feeding volumes, NEC incidence, or gastric residuals up to Day 7.

Ibuprofen is safer than indomethacin as it does not reduce mesenteric blood flow [29]. In a meta-analysis of 19 studies (956 infants), NEC rates were lower in the Ibuprofen group (typical RR 0.68 (95% CI 0.47, 0.99)) (LOE 1a) [30].

12. Assessment of Feed Tolerance

12.1. Suggestion

Do not check gastric residuals routinely. Check pre-feed gastric residual volume (GRV) only after a minimum feed volume (per feed) is attained. We suggest the following thresholds: <500 g: 2 mL, 500–749 g: 3 mL, 750–1000 g: 4 mL, >1000 g: 5 mL.

Do not check abdominal girth routinely.

Isolated green or yellow residuals are unimportant. Vomiting bile may indicate an intestinal obstruction or ileus. Withhold feeds in case of hemorrhagic residuals, as hemorrhagic residuals are significant.

12.2. Rationale

GRV is not as important a predictor of NEC as earlier thought. Below a certain feed volume, there is no point in checking the GRV. Among preterm babies on TPN, the mean + 2 SD value for GRV is about 4 mL (LOE 4) [31]. Mihatsch *et al.* [32] tolerated GRV up to 2 mL in infants <750 g and up to 3 mL in infants >750 g to 999 g. In a multiple regression model, the mean GRV and green residuals had no relationship with enteral feeding volume achieved by Day 14 (LOE 2b). In recent studies, ≤ 5 mL/kg has been used as a criterion for permissible GRV, but there are no comparisons between different cutoff values [33]. In a prospective study on 50 preterm infants, there was no correlation between feeding outcomes and GRV (mL/day) (LOE 2b) [34]. In a pilot RCT, 61 infants (24–32 weeks of gestation) were randomly allocated to receive routine evaluation of gastric residuals *versus* no routine evaluation [35]. There was no difference between the groups regarding volume of feeds at 3 weeks of age, growth, and days on TPN. Infants without routine evaluation of gastric residuals reached full feeds six days earlier.

In a case-control study on VLBWI with ($n = 17$) and without ($n = 17$) NEC, the mean maximum GRV as a percentage of the previous feed was 113% among subjects with NEC and 43% in controls (LOE 4) [36]. Hemorrhagic residuals, but not green residuals, were associated with NEC.

A study that suggested a relationship between modest GRV and NEC was a case-control study on 51 VLBWI with proven NEC and 102 healthy controls (LOE 4) [37]. The study was criticized for its choice of controls. There was a difference in the maximum GRV as a percentage of the corresponding feed volume between the NEC group and the controls (median (IQR): 40 (24, 61) *vs.* 14 (4, 33), $p < 0.001$), but with a large overlap between groups.

Although most studies have downplayed the importance of GRV, two retrospective studies, mentioned above, suggest there could be a relationship with NEC.

Green residuals could be due to duodenogastric reflux or overzealous aspiration, which could suck back duodenal contents (LOE 5) [38,39]. Studies have not found an association between green residuals and NEC (LOE 2b and 4) [32,36].

Abdominal girth is not a reliable measure of feed tolerance. There is a paucity of studies evaluating an increase in girth with clinical outcomes. It is highly prone to intra- and inter-observer variation. Abdominal circumference may vary by 3.5 cm during one feeding cycle in normal premature infants (LOE 4) [40]. It correlates with time from last defecation ($p = 0.0001$). Among term infants, the mean inter-observer difference is up to 1 cm [41].

13. Management of Residuals

13.1. Suggestion

Push back GRV of up to 5 mL/kg or 50% (whichever is higher) of the previous feed volume. If it recurs, subtract the residual volume from the current feed.

If the GRV is >5 mL/kg and >50% of the previous feed volume, push back the GRV up to 50% of the feed volume and do not give the current feed. If this happens again, consider slow bolus feeds or withholding feeds, depending on the clinical condition.

If the problem of residual volumes persists despite slow bolus feeds, consider decreasing the feed volume to the last well-tolerated feed volume.

Use the smallest volume syringe for checking residuals. Take care to aspirate gently.

After a feed, nurse the baby in the prone position for half an hour.

13.2. Rationale

The rationale for 5 mL/kg is covered in Section 11. The criterion of 50% is a round figure approximately equal to the cutoff from the study by Cobb *et al.* [37]. Pushing back partially digested gastric aspirates may replenish acid and enzymes that aid in the digestive process [42].

There is a paucity of data regarding the role of slow bolus feeding. In a physiologic study on pre-terms comparing a 120-min infusion of feeds compared to bolus feeds, the former was associated with faster gastric emptying, lower GRV, and more frequent duodenal motor responses (LOE 2b) [43]. Whether these theoretical advantages of slow bolus translate into clinical benefits is unclear, but there is a physiological basis for trying. In a Cochrane meta-analysis comparing continuous nasogastric *versus* intermittent bolus feeding in VLBWI, the continuous method resulted in a longer time to reach full enteral feeding (weighted mean difference (WMD) 3 days (95% CI 0.7, 5.2)), with no difference in growth or incidence of NEC (LOE 1a−) [44].

The narrower the diameter of the syringe, the less pressure is applied while pulling (as opposed to pushing) (LOE 4) [45]. Hence, smaller volume syringes are preferred.

In an RCT, the decrease in the volume of gastric residuals was lower in the prone position than in supine, and the rate of decrease of gastric residual volume was highest in the first half hour after the feed [46].

14. Clinical Diagnosis of Gastro-Esophageal Reflux (GER)

14.1. Suggestion

Do not rely on apnea, desaturation, or bradycardia; or behavioral signs, such as gagging, coughing, arching, and irritability, as signs of GER in preterm babies.

14.2. Rationale

The relationship between GER and cardio-respiratory events is controversial. Early studies either used a pH probe, which is unable to detect non-acid reflux; or used only the multi-channel intraluminal impedance (MII) probe, which underestimates acid GER events. The modality of choice is combined MII-pH monitoring.

In MII-pH studies on 71 preterm infants (mean birth weight 1319 g) there were 12,957 cardiorespiratory events and 4164 GER episodes, but GER preceded less than 3% of all cardiorespiratory events (LOE 2b) [47].

In another MII study on 19 preterm infants, the frequency of apneas occurring within 20 s of reflux episodes was not significantly different from that during reflux-free periods (LOE 2b) [48].

In a 24-h pH-MII study on 21 healthy premature infants, only 25% of reflux events were acidic [49]. Episodes that reached the proximal esophagus were also unassociated with cardio-respiratory events.

Contrary to the above, a group from Italy has published two reports using pH-MII monitoring that support the relationship between GER and apnea ≥ 5 s (LOE 2b) [50,51]. The frequency of apnea in the 30 s after GER was greater than in the 30 s before GER ($p = 0.01$). Apnea was shown to be associated with non-acid MII-GER episodes ($p = 0.000$), but not with acid GER episodes ($p = 0.137$).

We conclude that GER is probably not associated with cardio-respiratory events. At worst, it may cause brief episodes of apnea, and these are primarily from non-acidic episodes.

Snel *et al.* [52] studied 14 preterm infants (gestation of 26–35 weeks) who underwent continuous esophageal pH monitoring and videography (LOE 4). For each episode of acid GER, a 10-min video recording was analyzed and compared with a 10-min clipping when the esophageal pH exceeded 4. The recordings were randomized and viewed independently by two masked observers. There was no relationship between behavioral cues and reflux. The association of behavioral patterns with GER has only been reported in a study on eight term babies [53].

There is no difference in behavioral symptom scores after treatment with cisapride or omeprazole, emphasizing that they are possibly not because of GER (LOE 2b) [54,55].

15. Body Position for Treatment of GER

15.1. Suggestion

Place the baby in the left lateral position after a feed and turn over to the prone position about half an hour later. Elevate the head end to 30°. Place the infant supine for sleeping at home.

15.2. Rationale

Among 22 preterm infants with regurgitation who underwent 24-h recording of pH-MII in four body positions, the left lateral position showed the lowest esophageal acid exposure in the early post-prandial period and the prone position in the late post-prandial period (LOE 2b) [36].

Preterm infants are not an exception to the supine sleep recommendation for home care, because of the increased risk of sudden infant death syndrome (SIDS) among preterm infants [57,58].

16. Medications for Treatment of GER

16.1. Suggestion

Do not use domperidone, H2-blockers, or proton-pump inhibitors for the treatment of GER.

16.2. Rationale

In the only study evaluating domperidone, 13 infants with suspected GER treated with domperidone were compared to 13 untreated controls with suspected GER (LOE 2b) [59]. On 24-h pH-MII monitoring, the frequency of GER episodes was higher in the domperidone group ($p = 0.001$). A crossover trial on 18 infants comparing metoclopramide with a placebo had similar findings [60]. Domperidone is associated with prolongation of QTc interval in neonates above 32 weeks of gestation [61]. QTc prolongation has not been demonstrated in more premature infants ($n = 40$); however, we need additional data to declare domperidone as safe [62].

Ranitidine is associated with a higher incidence of late onset sepsis (LOE 4) [63] and NEC in preterm neonates (LOE 3b) [64]. In a study on VLBWI comparing $n = 91$ who had received ranitidine with $n = 183$ who had not, the odds of developing sepsis in the ranitidine group was 5.5-fold higher and of NEC 6.6-fold higher (LOE 2b) [65]. Mortality was also higher in neonates receiving ranitidine ($p = 0.003$).

In a double-blind placebo-controlled crossover study in preterm neonates, omeprazole reduced intra-gastric acidity but not the frequency of reflux symptoms (L4E 2b) [66]. In another double-blind RCT on 52 premature neonates with suspected GER, there were no differences between the esomeprazole and placebo groups with respect to percentage change from baseline in total number of signs and symptoms related to GER and number of reflux episodes [67].

The association of GER and cardio-respiratory events is itself questionable. The only study that shows an association concluded that it is with the non-acid reflux [51]. Observational data suggests that gastric acid suppression is associated with serious adverse events. Hence, there is little justification for pharmacological gastric acid suppression in the treatment of GER.

17. Thickening Feeds for GER

17.1. Suggestion

Avoid thickeners in the treatment of presumed GER.

17.2. Rationale

There are no RCTs evaluating the thickening of feeds in an exclusively neonatal population [68]. One non-randomized trial compared smectite in neonates with GER measured by 24-h pH monitoring (LOE 4) [69]. The use of open-label thickeners contaminated the groups. Postural therapy combined with smectite was followed by a decrease in GER ($p < 0.05$). In another non-randomized trial on 24 infants, a formula thickened with amylopectin did not decrease the incidence of GER-related apneas or apnea of prematurity [70]. There is no evidence to support the use of rice cereal or thickened formulae.

The safety of thickeners in preterm neonates is questionable. Xanthan gum-based, carob bean gum-based, and pectin-based thickeners have all been reported to cause NEC (LOE 4) [71–73].

18. Feed Duration and Route of Feeding for Treatment of GER

18.1. Suggestion

If one strongly suspects GER, and re-positioning does not help, one may increase the feed duration to 30–90 min. Make all attempts to reduce the duration back to a shorter duration as soon as possible. Use continuous or trans-pyloric feeding as a last resort for the management of GER and avoid them as far as possible. There is still insufficient evidence to recommend the use of erythromycin for the prevention or treatment of feed intolerance.

18.2. Rationale

The association of cardio-respiratory events with GER is itself questionable. Hence, the evaluation of any intervention to "treat" GER is fraught with problems. Altering feed duration and body position is probably less harmful than medications for GER.

The physiological benefits of slow gavage feeds have been described earlier (Section 12) [43]. However, in a cross-over RCT on 30 preterm infants who received 21 ± 1.5 mL/kg of milk per feed using bolus gavage feeding over 10 min or slow gavage feeding over 1 h, there was no difference in terms of frequency of apneas (>4 s), bradycardias, and desaturations (LOE 2b) [74]. The Cochrane meta-analysis comparing continuous nasogastric milk feeding *versus* intermittent bolus feeding in VLBWI has been described earlier (Section 12) [44].

In view of the above information, there may be limited justification for trying out slow enteral feeding but no justification for prolonged slow gavage feeds or continuous feeds.

A Cochrane review on nine RCTs of transpyloric *versus* gastric feeding in preterm infants concluded that transpyloric feeding did not improve feed tolerance or growth and had an increased risk for cessation of feeds and mortality (LOE 1a) [75]. Moreover, this review is not directly applicable because the trials were on transpyloric enteral feeding as an initial feeding strategy rather than as treatment for GER.

In a retrospective study on 72 VLBWI with apnea/bradycardia due to presumed GER, the authors observed a reduction in the average number of apnea/bradycardia episodes with transpyloric feeding ($p = 0.02$) (LOE 4) [76].

A Cochrane review on erythromycin (three prevention and seven treatment RCTs until 2007) included studies that varied in definition of feed intolerance and in the measurement, analysis, and reporting of outcomes [77]. Therefore, meta-analysis could not be done. Subsequently, in a placebo-controlled RCT on high-dose oral erythromycin (50 mg/kg/day), there was no significant difference reported in the time to reach full feeds [78]. Another RCT on the efficacy of intermediate-dose erythromycin in 45 VLBW infants >14 days of age with feed intolerance reported a significantly lower number of days to achieve full feeds (36.5 ± 7.4 days *versus* 54.7 ± 23.3 days; $p = 0.01$) and a lower number of days on TPN in the erythromycin group [79].

19. Prevention of Nutrient Loss during Slow Gavage or Continuous Feeds

19.1. Suggestion

Use the shortest possible extension tubing from the syringe to the baby to prevent nutrient loss. Do not draw up extra milk—other than that used for priming—into the syringe. If slow bolus feeds have to be used, keep the duration to a minimum.

19.2. Rationale

In an experimental study, continuous feeding resulted in (mean) 40% loss of fat, 33% of calcium, and 20% of phosphorus (LOE 2b) [80]. Infusion via gravity resulted in 6%, 9%, and 7% losses, respectively. Infusion by pump over 30 min resulted in intermediate losses. Fat adheres to the inner wall of the tubing, resulting in losses.

20. Human Milk Fortification

20.1. Suggestion

Start fortification when enteral intake reaches 100 mL/kg/day. Start at a concentration of 1:50 and if this is tolerated for 48 h increase to 1:25.

20.2. Rationale

Most authors have started human milk fortification at 100 mL/kg/day and at a concentration of 1:50 (LOE 5) [81–83]. In the only RCT that compared starting fortification with a human milk-based fortifier at 100 mL/kg/day *versus* starting at 40 mL/kg/day, there was no difference in outcomes (LOE 1b) [16]. However, it is unclear whether this can be extrapolated to a bovine milk-based fortifier. In a retrospective study on infants <31 weeks of gestation, the authors compared 53 infants who received HMF from the first feed with $n = 42$ who received it after reaching a feed volume of 50–100 mL/kg/day [84]. There were no differences in weight gain, but the early fortification group had a lower incidence of elevated alkaline phosphatase levels. Thus, more RCTs are required before recommending fortification at less than 100 mL/kg/day or an initial concentration less than 1:50.

21. Glycerin Enemas to Promote Feed Tolerance

21.1. Suggestion

Do not use daily glycerin suppositories to reduce the time to full enteral feeding. If one uses a trial of glycerin tips on a case-by-case basis, one should take into account the normal stooling pattern in preterm infants and volume of milk ingested to decide on the need for a glycerin tip.

21.2. Rationale

There is a relationship between gestation and the time of passage of the first stool: the lower the gestation, the longer the time taken [85].

In a study on 41 ELBW infants, there was an inverse correlation between feed volume on Day 14 and the last day of passing meconium but there was no correlation with the first day of passing (LOE 2b) [86]. In an observational study involving historical controls, VLBWI undergoing meconium evacuation by routine glycerin enema starting from Day 1 of life achieved full enteral feeding faster than controls (hazard ratio 2.9; 95% CI 1.8, 4.8) (LOE 2b) [87]. A subsequent RCT showed that daily glycerin suppositories did not reduce the time to full enteral feeding in infants born at less than 32 weeks of gestation (LOE 1b) [88]. Glycerin enemas may also cause rectal tears.

22. Conclusions

We suggest that physicians taking care of VLBW infants should aim to reach full feeds by about 2 weeks of age in neonates weighing <1000 g at birth and by about one week in neonates weighing 1000–1500 g at birth. A 3-hourly feeding regimen can be introduced for infants weighing >1250 g. Trophic feeds (10–15 mL/kg/day) should be started preferably within 24 h of life, but caution should be exercised in extremely preterm, ELBW or growth restricted infants. For babies weighing ≥1 kg at birth, we suggest starting nutritional feeds at 30 mL/kg/day and increase by 30 mL/kg/day. The first choice of milk is mother's own fresh milk. Among SGA infants with AREDF and a normal abdominal examination, feeding can be started within 24 h of life, and advanced cautiously. Feeds should be advanced cautiously in VLBW infants on non-invasive ventilation. If the neonate is already on minimal feeds, trophic feeds should be continued until the indomethacin course finishes. We advise against checking gastric residuals routinely. Abdominal girth should not be checked routinely. Isolated green or yellow residuals are unimportant. We suggest that GRV of 5 mL/kg or 50% (whichever is higher) of the previous feed volume should be pushed back and the amount subtracted from the current feed. One should not rely on apnea, desaturation or bradicardia; or behavioural signs as markers of GER in preterm babies. Body positioning in the left lateral or prone position may help with GER but medications and thickeners are not recommended. Slow gavage feeding may be attempted in GER after taking care to prevent nutrient losses. Human milk may be fortified after enteral intake of 100 mL/kg/day is reached. Glycerin enemas should not be used with the intention of reducing the time to full enteral feeding.

Author Contributions: Sourabh Dutta planned the review, supervised the search and critical appraisal of literature, wrote the first draft, and edited and approved the final draft submitted for publication. Balpreet Singh critically reviewed literature related to advancement of feeds, feed tolerance, continuous feeding, and donor milk; and contributed to the first draft of the manuscript. Lorraine Chessell critically reviewed literature related to trophic and nutritional feeds, gastric residuals, and fortification; and contributed to the first draft of the manuscript. Jennifer Wilson critically reviewed literature related to signs of feed intolerance and GER and contributed to the first draft of the manuscript. Marianne Janes critically reviewed literature related to rate of advancement, feed tolerance, and glycerin enemas; and contributed to the first draft of the manuscript. Kimberley McDonald critically reviewed literature related to type of milk and donor milk, and contributed to the first draft of the manuscript. Shaneela Shahid critically reviewed literature related to feeding in special circumstances and gastric residuals, and contributed to the first draft of the manuscript. Victoria A. Gardner critically reviewed literature related to feed tolerance and continuous feeding, and contributed to the first draft of the manuscript. Aune Hjartarson critically reviewed literature related to GER and contributed to the first draft of the manuscript. Margaret Purcha critically reviewed literature related to trophic feeding, nutritional feeds, and gastric residuals; and contributed to the first draft of the manuscript. Jennifer Watson critically reviewed literature related to median age to reach full feeds and signs of feed intolerance, and contributed to the first draft of the manuscript. Chris de Boer critically reviewed literature related to median age to reach full feeds and signs of feed intolerance, and contributed to the first draft of the manuscript. Barbara Gaal contributed to the first draft of the manuscript. Christoph Fusch conceptualized the need for the review, supervised the review process, and edited and approved the final manuscript as submitted.

Conflicts of Interest: The authors declare no conflict of interest.

References

1. Oxford Centre for Evidence-Based Medicine—Levels of Evidence (March 2009). Available online: http://www.cebm.net/oxford-centre-evidence-based-medicine-levels-evidence-march-2009/ (accessed on 1 January 2015).
2. Flidel-Rimon, O.; Friedman, S.; Lev, E.; Juster-Reicher, A.; Amitay, M.; Shinwell, E.S. Early enteral feeding and nosocomial sepsis in very low birthweight infants. *Arch. Dis. Child. Fetal Neonatal Ed.* **2004**, *89*, F289–F292. [CrossRef] [PubMed]
3. Hartel, C.; Haase, B.; Browning-Carmo, K.; Gebauer, C.; Kattner, E.; Kribs, A.; Segerer, H.; Teig, N.; Wense, A.; Wieg, C.; *et al.* Does the enteral feeding advancement affect short-term outcomes in very low birth weight infants? *J. Pediatr. Gastroenterol. Nutr.* **2009**, *48*, 464–470. [CrossRef] [PubMed]
4. Rochow, N.; Fusch, G.; Muhlinghaus, A.; Niesytto, C.; Straube, S.; Utzig, N.; Fusch, C. A nutritional program to improve outcome of very low birth weight infants. *Clin. Nutr.* **2012**, *31*, 124–131. [CrossRef] [PubMed]
5. McCallie, K.R.; Lee, H.C.; Mayer, O.; Cohen, R.S.; Hintz, S.R.; Rhine, W.D. Improved outcomes with a standardized feeding protocol for very low birth weight infants. *J. Perinatol.* **2011**, *31*, S61–S67. [CrossRef]
6. Krishnamurthy, S.; Gupta, P.; Debnath, S.; Gomber, S. Slow *versus* rapid enteral feeding advancement in preterm newborn infants 1000–1499 g: A randomized controlled trial. *Acta Paediatr.* **2010**, *99*, 42–46. [CrossRef] [PubMed]
7. Dhingra, A.; Agrawal, S.K.; Kumar, P.; Narang, A. A randomised controlled trial of two feeding schedules in neonates weighing ≤1750 g. *J. Matern. Fetal Neonatal Med.* **2009**, *22*, 198–203. [CrossRef] [PubMed]
8. Rudiger, M.; Herrmann, S.; Schmalisch, G.; Wauer, R.R.; Hammer, H.; Tschirch, E. Comparison of 2-h *versus* 3-h enteral feeding in extremely low birth weight infants, commencing after birth. *Acta Paediatr.* **2008**, *97*, 764–769. [CrossRef] [PubMed]
9. DeMauro, S.B.; Abbasi, S.; Lorch, S. The impact of feeding interval on feeding outcomes in very low birth-weight infants. *J. Perinatol.* **2011**, *31*, 481–486. [CrossRef] [PubMed]
10. Morgan, J.; Bombell, S.; McGuire, W. Early trophic feeding *versus* enteral fasting for very preterm or very low birth weight infants. *Cochrane Database Syst. Rev.* **2013**, *3*, CD000504. [CrossRef] [PubMed]
11. Dunn, L.; Hulman, S.; Weiner, J.; Kliegman, R. Beneficial effects of early hypocaloric enteral feeding on neonatal gastrointestinal function: Preliminary report of a randomized trial. *J. Pediatr.* **1988**, *112*, 622–629. [CrossRef] [PubMed]
12. Meetze, W.H.; Valentine, C.; McGuigan, J.E.; Conlon, M.; Sacks, N.; Neu, J. Gastrointestinal priming prior to full enteral nutrition in very low birth weight infants. *J. Pediatr. Gastroenterol. Nutr.* **1992**, *15*, 163–170. [CrossRef] [PubMed]
13. Morgan, J.; Young, L.; McGuire, W. Delayed introduction of progressive enteral feeds to prevent necrotising enterocolitis in very low birth weight infants. *Cochrane Database Syst. Rev.* **2014**, *12*, CD001970. [CrossRef] [PubMed]
14. Morgan, J.; Young, L.; McGuire, W. Slow advancement of enteral feed volumes to prevent necrotising enterocolitis in very low birth weight infants. *Cochrane Database Syst. Rev.* **2014**, *12*, CD001241. [CrossRef] [PubMed]
15. Schanler, R.J. Outcomes of human milk-fed premature infants. *Semin. Perinatol.* **2011**, *35*, 29–33. [CrossRef] [PubMed]
16. Sullivan, S.; Schanler, R.J.; Kim, J.H.; Patel, A.L.; Trawoger, R.; Kiechl-Kohlendorfer, U.; Chan, G.M.; Blanco, C.L.; Abrams, S.; Cotten, C.M.; *et al.* An exclusively human milk-based diet is associated with a lower rate of necrotizing enterocolitis than a diet of human milk and bovine milk-based products. *J. Pediatr.* **2010**, *156*, 562–567. [CrossRef] [PubMed]

17. Cristofalo, E.A.; Schanler, R.J.; Blanco, C.L.; Sullivan, S.; Trawoeger, R.; Kiechl-Kohlendorfer, U.; Dudell, G.; Rechtman, D.J.; Lee, M.L.; Lucas, A.; *et al.* Randomized trial of exclusive human milk *versus* preterm formula diets in extremely premature infants. *J. Pediatr.* **2013**, *163*, 1592–1595. [CrossRef] [PubMed]

18. Schanler, R.J.; Lau, C.; Hurst, N.M.; Smith, E.O. Randomized trial of donor human milk *versus* preterm formula as substitutes for mothers' own milk in the feeding of extremely premature infants. *Pediatrics* **2005**, *116*, 400–406. [CrossRef] [PubMed]

19. Ganapathy, V.; Hay, J.W.; Kim, J.H. Costs of necrotizing enterocolitis and cost-effectiveness of exclusively human milk-based products in feeding extremely premature infants. *Breastfeed. Med.* **2012**, *7*, 29–37. [CrossRef] [PubMed]

20. Mihatsch, W.A.; Pohlandt, F.; Franz, A.R.; Flock, F. Early feeding advancement in very-low-birth-weight infants with intrauterine growth retardation and increased umbilical artery resistance. *J. Pediatr. Gastroenterol. Nutr.* **2002**, *35*, 144–148. [CrossRef] [PubMed]

21. Karagianni, P.; Briana, D.D.; Mitsiakos, G.; Elias, A.; Theodoridis, T.; Chatziioannidis, E.; Kyriakidou, M.; Nikolaidis, N. Early *versus* delayed minimal enteral feeding and risk for necrotizing enterocolitis in preterm growth-restricted infants with abnormal antenatal Doppler results. *Am. J. Perinatol.* **2010**, *27*, 367–373. [CrossRef] [PubMed]

22. Van Elburg, R.M.; van den Berg, A.; Bunkers, C.M.; van Lingen, R.A.; Smink, E.W.; van, E.J.; Fetter, W.P. Minimal enteral feeding, fetal blood flow pulsatility, and postnatal intestinal permeability in preterm infants with intrauterine growth retardation. *Arch. Dis. Child. Fetal Neonatal Ed.* **2004**, *89*, F293–F296. [PubMed]

23. Leaf, A.; Dorling, J.; Kempley, S.; McCormick, K.; Mannix, P.; Linsell, L.; Juszczak, E.; Brocklehurst, P. Early or delayed enteral feeding for preterm growth-restricted infants: A randomized trial. *Pediatrics* **2012**, *129*, e1260–e1268. [CrossRef] [PubMed]

24. Kempley, S.; Gupta, N.; Linsell, L.; Dorling, J.; McCormick, K.; Mannix, P.; Juszczak, E.; Brocklehurst, P.; Leaf, A. Feeding infants below 29 weeks' gestation with abnormal antenatal Doppler: Analysis from a randomised trial. *Arch. Dis. Child. Fetal Neonatal Ed.* **2014**, *99*, F6–F11. [PubMed]

25. Havranek, T.; Madramootoo, C.; Carver, J.D. Nasal continuous positive airway pressure affects pre- and postprandial intestinal blood flow velocity in preterm infants. *J. Perinatol.* **2007**, *27*, 704–708. [CrossRef] [PubMed]

26. Jaile, J.C.; Levin, T.; Wung, J.T.; Abramson, S.J.; Ruzal-Shapiro, C.; Berdon, W.E. Benign gaseous distension of the bowel in premature infants treated with nasal continuous airway pressure: A study of contributing factors. *Am. J. Roentgenol.* **1992**, *158*, 125–127. [CrossRef]

27. Clyman, R.; Wickremasinghe, A.; Jhaveri, N.; Hassinger, D.C.; Attridge, J.T.; Sanocka, U.; Polin, R.; Gillam-Krakauer, M.; Reese, J.; Mammel, M.; *et al.* Enteral feeding during indomethacin and ibuprofen treatment of a patent ductus arteriosus. *J. Pediatr.* **2013**, *163*, 406–411. [CrossRef] [PubMed]

28. Bellander, M.; Ley, D.; Polberger, S.; Hellstrom-Westas, L. Tolerance to early human milk feeding is not compromised by indomethacin in preterm infants with persistent ductus arteriosus. *Acta Paediatr.* **2003**, *92*, 1074–1078. [CrossRef] [PubMed]

29. Pezzati, M.; Vangi, V.; Biagiotti, R.; Bertini, G.; Cianciulli, D.; Rubaltelli, F.F. Effects of indomethacin and ibuprofen on mesenteric and renal blood flow in preterm infants with patent ductus arteriosus. *J. Pediatr.* **1999**, *135*, 733–738. [CrossRef] [PubMed]

30. Ohlsson, A.; Walia, R.; Shah, S.S. Ibuprofen for the treatment of patent ductus arteriosus in preterm and/or low birth weight infants. *Cochrane Database Syst Rev.* **2013**, *4*, CD003481. [CrossRef] [PubMed]

31. Malhotra, A.K.; Deorari, A.K.; Paul, V.K.; Bagga, A.; Singh, M. Gastric residuals in preterm babies. *J. Trop. Pediatr.* **1992**, *38*, 262–264. [CrossRef] [PubMed]

32. Mihatsch, W.A.; von Schoenaich, P.; Fahnenstich, H.; Dehne, N.; Ebbecke, H.; Plath, C.; von Stockhausen, H.B.; Muche, R.; Franz, A.; Pohlandt, F. The significance of gastric residuals in the early enteral feeding advancement of extremely low birth weight infants. *Pediatrics* **2002**, *109*, 457–459. [CrossRef] [PubMed]

33. Mihatsch, W.A.; Franz, A.R.; Hogel, J.; Pohlandt, F. Hydrolyzed protein accelerates feeding advancement in very low birth weight infants. *Pediatrics* **2002**, *110*, 1199–1203. [CrossRef] [PubMed]

34. Shulman, R.J.; Ou, C.N.; Smith, E.O. Evaluation of potential factors predicting attainment of full gavage feedings in preterm infants. *Neonatology* **2011**, *99*, 38–44. [CrossRef] [PubMed]

35. Torrazza, R.M.; Parker, L.A.; Talaga, E.; Shuster, J.; Neu, J. The value of routine evaluation of gastric residuals in very low birth weight infants. *J. Perinatol.* **2014**. [CrossRef]

36. Bertino, E.; Giuliani, F.; Prandi, G.; Coscia, A.; Martano, C.; Fabris, C. Necrotizing enterocolitis: Risk factor analysis and role of gastric residuals in very low birth weight infants. *J. Pediatr. Gastroenterol. Nutr.* **2009**, *48*, 437–442. [CrossRef] [PubMed]

37. Cobb, B.A.; Carlo, W.A.; Ambalavanan, N. Gastric residuals and their relationship to necrotizing enterocolitis in very low birth weight infants. *Pediatrics* **2004**, *113*, 50–53. [CrossRef] [PubMed]

38. Eizaguirre, I.; Emparanza, J.; Tovar, J.A.; Weilin, W.; Tapia, I. Duodenogastric reflux: Values in normal children and in children with gastroesophageal reflux. *Cir. Pediatr.* **1993**, *6*, 114–116. (In Spanish) [PubMed]

39. Wang, W.; Ji, S.; Wang, H.; Wang, W. 24-Hour gastroesophageal double pH monitoring acid and alkaline gastroesophageal and duodenogastric refluxes in pediatric patients. *Chin. Med. J. (Engl.)* **1998**, *111*, 881–884.

40. Bhatia, P.; Johnson, K.J.; Bell, E.F. Variability of abdominal circumference of premature infants. *J. Pediatr. Surg.* **1990**, *25*, 543–544. [CrossRef] [PubMed]

41. Johnson, T.S.; Engstrom, J.L.; Gelhar, D.K. Intra- and interexaminer reliability of anthropometric measurements of term infants. *J. Pediatr. Gastroenterol. Nutr.* **1997**, *24*, 497–505. [CrossRef] [PubMed]

42. Li, Y.; Lin, H.; Torrazza, R.M.; Parker, L.; Talaga, E.; Neu, J. Gastric residual evaluation in preterm neonates: A useful monitoring technique or a hindrance? *Pediatr. Neonatol.* **2014**, *55*, 335–340. [CrossRef] [PubMed]

43. De, V.K.; Knapp, E.; Al-Tawil, Y.; Berseth, C.L. Slow infusion feedings enhance duodenal motor responses and gastric emptying in preterm infants. *Am. J. Clin. Nutr.* **1998**, *68*, 103–108. [PubMed]

44. Premji, S.; Chessell, L. Continuous nasogastric milk feeding *versus* intermittent bolus milk feeding for premature infants less than 1500 grams. *Cochrane Database Syst Rev.* **2011**, *11*, CD001819. [CrossRef] [PubMed]

45. Macklin, D. What's physics got to do with it? A review of the physical principles of fluid administration. *J. Vasc. Access Devices* **1999**, *4*, 7–11. [CrossRef]

46. Chen, S.S.; Tzeng, Y.L.; Gau, B.S.; Kuo, P.C.; Chen, J.Y. Effects of prone and supine positioning on gastric residuals in preterm infants: A time series with cross-over study. *Int. J. Nurs. Stud.* **2013**, *50*, 1459–1467. [CrossRef] [PubMed]

47. Di, F.J.; Arko, M.; Herynk, B.; Martin, R.; Hibbs, A.M. Characterization of cardiorespiratory events following gastroesophageal reflux in preterm infants. *J. Perinatol.* **2010**, *30*, 683–687. [CrossRef] [PubMed]

48. Peter, C.S.; Sprodowski, N.; Bohnhorst, B.; Silny, J.; Poets, C.F. Gastroesophageal reflux and apnea of prematurity: No temporal relationship. *Pediatrics* **2002**, *109*, 8–11. [CrossRef] [PubMed]

49. Lopez-Alonso, M.; Moya, M.J.; Cabo, J.A.; Ribas, J.; del Carmen, M.M.; Silny, J.; Sifrim, D. Twenty-four-hour esophageal impedance-pH monitoring in healthy preterm neonates: Rate and characteristics of acid, weakly acidic, and weakly alkaline gastroesophageal reflux. *Pediatrics* **2006**, *118*, e299–e308. [CrossRef] [PubMed]

50. Corvaglia, L.; Zama, D.; Gualdi, S.; Ferlini, M.; Aceti, A.; Faldella, G. Gastro-oesophageal reflux increases the number of apnoeas in very preterm infants. *Arch. Dis. Child. Fetal Neonatal Ed.* **2009**, *94*, F188–F192. [CrossRef] [PubMed]

51. Corvaglia, L.; Zama, D.; Spizzichino, M.; Aceti, A.; Mariani, E.; Capretti, M.G.; Galletti, S.; Faldella, G. The frequency of apneas in very preterm infants is increased after non-acid gastro-esophageal reflux. *Neurogastroenterol. Motil.* **2011**, *23*, 303–307, e152. [CrossRef] [PubMed]

52. Snel, A.; Barnett, C.P.; Cresp, T.L.; Haslam, R.R.; Davidson, G.P.; Malbert, T.H.; Dent, J.; Omari, T.I. Behavior and gastroesophageal reflux in the premature neonate. *J. Pediatr. Gastroenterol. Nutr.* **2000**, *30*, 18–21. [CrossRef] [PubMed]

53. Feranchak, A.P.; Orenstein, S.R.; Cohn, J.F. Behaviors associated with onset of gastroesophageal reflux episodes in infants. Prospective study using split-screen video and pH probe. *Clin. Pediatr. (Phila.)* **1994**, *33*, 654–662. [CrossRef]

54. Barnett, C.P.; Omari, T.; Davidson, G.P.; Goodchild, L.; Lontis, R.; Dent, J.; Haslam, R.R. Effect of cisapride on gastric emptying in premature infants with feed intolerance. *J. Paediatr. Child Health* **2001**, *37*, 559–563. [CrossRef] [PubMed]

55. Moore, D.J.; Tao, B.S.; Lines, D.R.; Hirte, C.; Heddle, M.L.; Davidson, G.P. Double-blind placebo-controlled trial of omeprazole in irritable infants with gastroesophageal reflux. *J. Pediatr.* **2003**, *143*, 219–223. [CrossRef] [PubMed]

56. Corvaglia, L.; Rotatori, R.; Ferlini, M.; Aceti, A.; Ancora, G.; Faldella, G. The effect of body positioning on gastroesophageal reflux in premature infants: Evaluation by combined impedance and pH monitoring. *J. Pediatr.* **2007**, *151*, 591–596. [CrossRef] [PubMed]

57. American Academy of Pediatrics. Task force on sudden infant death syndrome. The changing concept of sudden infant death syndrome: Diagnostic coding shifts, controversies regarding the sleeping environment, and new variables to consider in reducing risk. *Pediatrics* **2005**, *116*, 1245–1255.

58. Canadian Pediatric Society. Recommendations for Safe Sleeping Environments for Infants and Children. *Paediatr. Child Health.* **2004**, *9*, 659–663.

59. Cresi, F.; Marinaccio, C.; Russo, M.C.; Miniero, R.; Silvestro, L. Short-term effect of domperidone on gastroesophageal reflux in newborns assessed by combined intraluminal impedance and pH monitoring. *J. Perinatol.* **2008**, *28*, 766–770. [CrossRef] [PubMed]

60. Wheatley, E.; Kennedy, K.A. Cross-over trial of treatment for bradycardia attributed to gastroesophageal reflux in preterm infants. *J. Pediatr.* **2009**, *155*, 516–521. [CrossRef] [PubMed]

61. Djeddi, D.; Kongolo, G.; Lefaix, C.; Mounard, J.; Leke, A. Effect of domperidone on QT interval in neonates. *J. Pediatr.* **2008**, *153*, 663–666. [CrossRef] [PubMed]

62. Gunlemez, A.; Babaoglu, A.; Arisoy, A.E.; Turker, G.; Gokalp, A.S. Effect of domperidone on the QTc interval in premature infants. *J. Perinatol.* **2010**, *30*, 50–53. [CrossRef] [PubMed]

63. Bianconi, S.; Gudavalli, M.; Sutija, V.G.; Lopez, A.L.; Barillas-Arias, L.; Ron, N. Ranitidine and late-onset sepsis in the neonatal intensive care unit. *J. Perinat. Med.* **2007**, *35*, 147–150. [CrossRef] [PubMed]

64. Guillet, R.; Stoll, B.J.; Cotten, C.M.; Gantz, M.; McDonald, S.; Poole, W.K.; Phelps, D.L. Association of H2-blocker therapy and higher incidence of necrotizing enterocolitis in very low birth weight infants. *Pediatrics* **2006**, *117*, e137–e142. [CrossRef] [PubMed]

65. Terrin, G.; Passariello, A.; De, C.M.; Manguso, F.; Salvia, G.; Lega, L.; Messina, F.; Paludetto, R.; Canani, R.B. Ranitidine is associated with infections, necrotizing enterocolitis, and fatal outcome in newborns. *Pediatrics* **2012**, *129*, e40–e45. [CrossRef] [PubMed]

66. Omari, T.I.; Haslam, R.R.; Lundborg, P.; Davidson, G.P. Effect of omeprazole on acid gastroesophageal reflux and gastric acidity in preterm infants with pathological acid reflux. *J. Pediatr. Gastroenterol. Nutr.* **2007**, *44*, 41–44. [CrossRef] [PubMed]

67. Davidson, G.; Wenzl, T.G.; Thomson, M.; Omari, T.; Barker, P.; Lundborg, P.; Illueca, M. Efficacy and safety of once-daily esomeprazole for the treatment of gastroesophageal reflux disease in neonatal patients. *J. Pediatr.* **2013**, *163*, 692–698. [CrossRef] [PubMed]

68. Huang, R.C.; Forbes, D.; Davies, M.W. Feed thickener for newborn infants with gastro-oesophageal reflux. *Cochrane Database Syst. Rev.* **2002**, *3*, CD003211. [CrossRef] [PubMed]

69. Gouyon, J.B.; Boggio, V.; Fantino, M.; Gillot, I.; Schatz, B.; Vallin, A. Smectite reduces gastroesophageal reflux in newborn infants. *Dev. Pharmacol. Ther.* **1989**, *13*, 46–50. [PubMed]

70. Corvaglia, L.; Spizzichino, M.; Aceti, A.; Legnani, E.; Mariani, E.; Martini, S.; Battistini, B.; Faldella, G. A thickened formula does not reduce apneas related to gastroesophageal reflux in preterm infants. *Neonatology* **2013**, *103*, 98–102. [CrossRef] [PubMed]

71. Woods, C.W.; Oliver, T.; Lewis, K.; Yang, Q. Development of necrotizing enterocolitis in premature infants receiving thickened feeds using SimplyThick®. *J. Perinatol.* **2012**, *32*, 150–152. [CrossRef] [PubMed]

72. Clarke, P.; Robinson, M.J. Thickening milk feeds may cause necrotising enterocolitis. *Arch. Dis. Child. Fetal Neonatal Ed.* **2004**, *89*, F280. [CrossRef] [PubMed]

73. Mercier, J.C.; Hartmann, J.F.; Cohen, R.; Tran, H.; Biriotti, V.; Kessler, A. Intestinal occlusion and enterocolitis caused by Gelopectose. *Arch. Fr. Pediatr.* **1984**, *41*, 709–710. (In French) [PubMed]

74. Poets, C.F.; Langner, M.U.; Bohnhorst, B. Effects of bottle feeding and two different methods of gavage feeding on oxygenation and breathing patterns in preterm infants. *Acta Paediatr.* **1997**, *86*, 419–423. [CrossRef] [PubMed]

75. Watson, J.; McGuire, W. Transpyloric *versus* gastric tube feeding for preterm infants. *Cochrane Database Syst. Rev.* **2013**, *2*, CD003487. [CrossRef] [PubMed]

76. Malcolm, W.F.; Smith, P.B.; Mears, S.; Goldberg, R.N.; Cotten, C.M. Transpyloric tube feeding in very low birthweight infants with suspected gastroesophageal reflux: Impact on apnea and bradycardia. *J. Perinatol.* **2009**, *29*, 372–375. [CrossRef] [PubMed]

77. Ng, E.; Shah, V.S. Erythromycin for the prevention and treatment of feeding intolerance in preterm infants. *Cochrane Database Syst. Rev.* **2008**, *3*, CD001815. [CrossRef] [PubMed]

78. Mansi, Y.; Abdelaziz, N.; Ezzeldin, Z.; Ibrahim, R. Randomized controlled trial of a high dose of oral erythromycin for the treatment of feeding intolerance in preterm infants. *Neonatology* **2011**, *100*, 290–294. [CrossRef] [PubMed]

79. Ng, Y.; Su, P.; Chen, J.; Quek, Y.; Hu, J.; Lee, I.; Lee, H.; Chang, H. Efficacy of intermediate-dose oral erythromycin on very low birth weight infants with feeding intolerance. *Pediatr. Neonatol.* **2012**, *53*, 34–40. [CrossRef] [PubMed]

80. Rogers, S.P.; Hicks, P.D.; Hamzo, M.; Veit, L.E.; Abrams, S.A. Continuous feedings of fortified human milk deeds to nutrient losses of fat, calcium and phosphorus. *Nutrients* **2010**, *2*, 230–240. [CrossRef] [PubMed]

81. Berseth, C.L.; Van Aerde, J.E.; Gross, S.; Stolz, S.I.; Harris, C.L.; Hansen, J.W. Growth, efficacy, and safety of feeding an iron-fortified human milk fortifier. *Pediatrics* **2004**, *114*, e699–e706. [CrossRef] [PubMed]

82. Schanler, R.J.; Abrams, S.A. Postnatal attainment of intrauterine macromineral accretion rates in low birth weight infants fed fortified human milk. *J. Pediatr.* **1995**, *126*, 441–447. [CrossRef] [PubMed]

83. Schanler, R.J.; Shulman, R.J.; Lau, C. Feeding strategies for premature infants: Beneficial outcomes of feeding fortified human milk *versus* preterm formula. *Pediatrics* **1999**, *103*, 1150–1157. [CrossRef] [PubMed]

84. Tillman, S.; Brandon, D.H.; Silva, S.G. Evaluation of human milk fortification from the time of the first feeding: Effects on infants of less than 31 weeks gestational age. *J. Perinatol.* **2012**, *32*, 525–531. [CrossRef] [PubMed]

85. Weaver, L.T.; Lucas, A. Development of bowel habit in preterm infants. *Arch. Dis. Child.* **1993**, *68*, 317–320. [CrossRef] [PubMed]

86. Mihatsch, W.A.; Franz, A.R.; Lindner, W.; Pohlandt, F. Meconium passage in extremely low birthweight infants and its relation to very early enteral nutrition. *Acta Paediatr.* **2001**, *90*, 409–411. [CrossRef] [PubMed]

87. Shim, S.Y.; Kim, H.S.; Kim, D.H.; Kim, E.K.; Son, D.W.; Kim, B.I.; Choi, J.H. Induction of early meconium evacuation promotes feeding tolerance in very low birth weight infants. *Neonatology* **2007**, *92*, 67–72. [CrossRef] [PubMed]

88. Khadr, S.N.; Ibhanesebhor, S.E.; Rennix, C.; Fisher, H.E.; Manjunatha, C.M.; Young, D.; Abara, R.C. Randomized controlled trial: Impact of glycerin suppositories on time to full feeds in preterm infants. *Neonatology* **2011**, *100*, 169–176. [CrossRef] [PubMed]

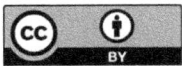

nutrients

MDPI

Article

Fortifier and Cream Improve Fat Delivery in Continuous Enteral Infant Feeding of Breast Milk

Mika Tabata [1],*, Khaled Abdelrahman [2], Amy B. Hair [3], Keli M. Hawthorne [3], Zhensheng Chen [3] and Steven A. Abrams [3]

[1] Department of Bioengineering, Rice University, 6100 Main St., Houston, TX 77005, USA
[2] Department of Bioengineering, University of Pittsburgh, 4200 Fifth Ave., Pittsburgh, PA 15260, USA; kha9@pitt.edu
[3] Children's Nutrition Research Center, Department of Agriculture/Agriculture Research Service, Department of Pediatrics, United States Baylor College of Medicine and Texas Children's Hospital, 1100 Bates Ave., Houston, TX 77030, USA; abhair@bcm.edu (A.B.H.); kelih@bcm.edu (K.M.H.); zchen1@bcm.edu (Z.C.); sabrams@bcm.edu (S.A.A.)
* Author to whom correspondence should be addressed; tabata@alumni.rice.edu; Tel.: +713-560-8225.

Received: 27 November 2014; Accepted: 26 January 2015; Published: 11 February 2015

Abstract: Premature and high-risk infants require accurate delivery of nutrients to promote appropriate growth. Continuous enteral feeding methods may result in significant fat and micronutrient loss. This study evaluated fat loss in enteral nutrition using current strategies for providing high-risk infants fortified human milk (HM). The fat content of HM was measured by IR analyzer in a simulated feeding system using the Kangaroo ePump™ and the MedFusion™ 2010 pump. Comparisons in fat loss were made between HM, HM supplemented with donor HM-derived fortifier Prolacta + H^2MF™ (H^2MF), and HM supplemented with H^2MF and donor HM-derived cream ProlactCR™ (cream). When using the Kangaroo ePump™, the addition of H^2MF and cream to HM increased fat delivery efficiency from 75.0% ± 1.2% to 83.7% ± 1.0% ($p < 0.0001$). When using the MedFusion™ 2010 pump, the addition of H^2MF to HM increased fat delivery efficiency from 83.2% ± 2.8% to 88.8% ± 0.8% ($p < 0.05$), and the addition of H^2MF and cream increased fat delivery efficiency to 92.0% ± 0.3% ($p < 0.01$). The addition of H^2MF and cream to HM provides both the benefits of bioactive elements from mother's milk and increased fat delivery, making the addition of H^2MF and cream an appropriate method to improve infant weight gain.

Keywords: enteral nutrition; breast milk; human milk-derived fortifier; human milk-derived cream supplement; very low birth weight; neonates; Kangaroo ePump™; MedFusion™ pump; neonatal intensive care units

---

1. Introduction

Very low birth weight (VLBW) and other high-risk infants require accurate delivery of nutrients in order to optimally grow during their hospital stay. The current feeding methods include syringe, bolus, and pump feeding. Human milk (HM) provides a wide range of benefits due to bioactive elements [1]. However, as previously shown [2–6], substantial amounts of fat and nutrients are lost throughout the delivery of HM by continuous syringe and pump feeding methods, due to fat adherence to the feeding bag, syringe and tubing. This fat adherence has been visually observed in previous studies [5]. Furthermore, limited assessment of the nutrients that reach the infant has been performed [7]. While minimal fat and nutrients from HM are lost through bolus feeding, many VLBW infants cannot tolerate the high flow rates required for bolus feeding.

The Kangaroo ePump™ and MedFusion™ syringe pumps are prevalent in many neonatal intensive care units (NICUs), although a substantial amount of phosphorus, calcium, and other nutrients that bind to fat are lost in these delivery processes when used for continuous feedings [5]. When mother's milk contains inadequate fat levels, many NICUs either replace HM with formula, which is not affected by fat adherence to tubing but does not contain bioactive elements found in HM, or add fortifiers such as HM-derived fortifier Prolacta + H^2MF^{TM} (H^2MF) with or without donor HM-derived cream ProlactCR™ (cream) to HM to increase the fat content. ProlactCR™ cream is a pasteurized donor HM-derived fat from HM which yields 2.5 calories·mL^{-1} and is intended as a supplement for mother's own milk or donor HM in order to provide the infant with an exclusively HM-based diet. Evidence shows that an exclusively HM-based diet is associated with significantly lower rates of necrotizing enterocolitis (NEC) and surgical NEC when compared with preterm formula and with a mother's milk-based diet supplemented with bovine milk–based products [8,9]. Furthermore, an exclusive HM-based diet is associated with lower mortality and morbidity in extremely preterm infants [10].

In order to improve the growth rate of premature and other high-risk infants, evaluations must be conducted to determine fat and nutrient losses due to different feeding methods and how it may be feasible to minimize these losses. The objective of this study was to evaluate fat loss in enteral nutrition using current strategies for delivering fortified HM to high-risk infants. We explore the use of HM-derived fortifier and cream to improve fat delivery efficiency, making it possible to deliver the bioactive elements of HM while increasing fat delivery to infants.

2. Experimental Section

2.1. Human Milk Sample Preparation

All HM used in this study was obtained through the mother's milk bank of Texas Children's Hospital in Houston, Texas and was designated for research purposes. HM from five anonymous mothers was pooled into a 4 L container, separated into aliquots in 50 mL VWR™ conical tubes, and stored in a freezer at $-20°C$. Before testing, HM was thawed with warm water and agitated using a common lab vortexer at 500 rpm to ensure homogeneity of the HM. No HM was used that had been thawed for over 24 h, which is the limit used by lactation services in the Texas Children's Hospital NICU for feeding infants.

HM with H^2MF was prepared by mixing 20 mL of H^2MF with 80 mL of HM, resulting in a 1:4 ratio of H^2MF to HM. HM with H^2MF and cream was prepared by combining 8 mL of cream with 20 mL of H^2MF and 80 mL of HM, resulting in a 2:5:20 ratio of cream to H^2MF to HM. These ratios follow clinical guidelines for HM containing 15–15.9 kcal·oz^{-1} [11]. Although the average energy content of HM is approximately 20 kcal·oz^{-1}, there is great variability, and in the United States, values have been reported ranging from 13.8 kcal·oz^{-1} to 25.1 kcal·oz^{-1} with 51% of HM having less than 19.2 kcal·oz^{-1} [12]. Fortification is recommended for HM containing less than 20 kcal·oz^{-1} [11]. Thus, adding fortifier and cream in the ratio for HM containing 15–15.9 kcal·oz^{-1} presumes the HM has a mid-range energy content of HM requiring fortification.

2.2. Experimental Setup/Feeding Simulations

All experiments in this study were conducted using a simulated continuous enteral feeding system, representing a typical NICU enteral feeding setup with variations between simulating feedings only in pump type and milk given. Variations of HM tested were HM, HM + H^2MF, and HM + H^2MF + cream. All simulated feedings used either the MedFusion 2010™ or the Kangaroo ePump™.

Before starting simulated feeds, 5 mL aliquots of HM were collected in 15 mL VWR™ tubes and processed for analysis of fat content directly thereafter, representing a "pre-feeding" aliquot.

The Kangaroo ePump™ was set up as it would be in typical NICU procedures. The bag (1000 mL Kangaroo ePump™ enteral pump set) was set 18 inches directly above the pump, and the collection site was level with the pump. The MedFusion™ pump was set up in the horizontal position and used with Monoject 35 mL syringes, which are made of polypropylene. Simulated feeds using the MedFusion™

pump were given through Covidien 60ES tubing extensions, which are made of polyvinyl chloride. Simulated feeds using the Kangaroo ePump™ were given through Kangaroo ePump™ 1000 mL Pump Sets (part #773656), which are made of polyvinyl chloride.

All simulated feeds were given at a flow rate of 20 mL·h^{-1} for 60 min. Aliquots at 5, 10, 15, 30, 45, and 60 min after the start of the feed were collected in 15 mL VWR™ tubes and were processed for analysis of fat content directly after collection.

2.3. Human Milk Sample Analysis

Prior to analysis, samples were warmed to 25–33 °C and homogenized using a probe sonicator (Q55 sonicator; Misonix Qsonica, Newton, Connecticut) for 10 s. HM samples were analyzed for fat concentration (g·mL^{-1}) and energy content (kcal·oz^{-1}) using a near-infrared milk analyzer (sample volume of 2 mL, Spectrastar™; Unity Scientific, Brookfield, Connecticut), following the Unity Scientific Procedure for Analyzing Breast Milk. For each milk sample, the average of three readings from the milk analyzer was recorded. The Spectrastar™ has been shown to measure fat content precisely but has room for improvement in accuracy [13].

2.4. Statistical Analysis

Total mass of fat as well as energy delivered throughout the entire duration of the simulated feed were calculated by right-handed integral approximation. The percentages of these approximations compared to the baseline fat content ("pre" feeding) integrated over the length of the feed represent the overall fat delivery efficiency. Data was analyzed using StatPlus®mac: LE (Copyright © 2010). Unpaired Student's *t*-tests assuming unequal variances were performed to determine statistically significant differences between fat delivery efficiencies of these categories of HM. Statistical significance was reached if $p < 0.05$.

3. Results

The addition of H^{2}MF to HM affected overall fat delivery efficiency when the MedFusion™ pump was used but not when the Kangaroo ePump™ was used. When the Kangaroo ePump™ was used, simulated feeds with HM produced an overall fat delivery efficiency of 75.0 ± 1.2%, while simulated feeds with HM + H^{2}MF produced an overall fat delivery efficiency of 75.9 ± 1.1% (Table 1). Thus, no significant difference in fat delivery efficiency was observed with the addition of H^{2}MF to HM when using the Kangaroo ePump™ ($p > 0.05$). However, when the MedFusion™ pump was used, simulated feeds with HM produced an overall fat delivery efficiency of 83.2 ± 2.8%, while simulated feeds with HM + H^{2}MF produced an overall fat delivery efficiency of 88.8 ± 0.8% (Table 1). Thus, a significant increase in fat delivery efficiency was observed with the addition of H^{2}MF to HM when using the MedFusion™ pump ($p < 0.05$).

Table 1. Fat delivery efficiency of HM, HM + H^{2}MF, and HM + H^{2}MF + cream.

	HM	HM + H^{2}MF	HM + H^{2}MF + cream
Kangaroo ePump™	75.0% ± 1.2% ($n = 8$)	75.9% ± 1.1% ($n = 8$)	83.7 ± 1.0% ($n = 8$) *
MedFusion™	83.2% ± 2.8% ($n = 9$)	88.8% ± 0.8% ($n = 6$) *	92.0 ± 0.3% ($n = 6$) *

* Denotes statistical significance compared to corresponding simulated feed with HM; HM: human milk; H^{2}MF: HM supplemented with donor HM-derived fortifier Prolacta + H^{2}MF™; Cream: HM supplemented with H^{2}MF and donor HM-derived cream ProlactCR™.

The addition of H^{2}MF and cream to HM increased the overall fat delivery efficiency of both pumps. When the Kangaroo ePump™ was used, simulated feeds with HM + H^{2}MF + cream resulted in an overall fat delivery efficiency of 83.7 ± 1.0%, compared to 75.0 ± 1.2% when HM alone was provided ($p < 0.0001$) and to 75.9 ± 1.1% when HM+H^{2}MF was provided ($p < 0.0001$) (Table 1). When the MedFusion™ pump was used, simulated feeds with HM + H^{2}MF + cream resulted in an overall fat delivery efficiency of $92.0 \pm 0.3\%$, compared to $83.2 \pm 2.8\%$ when HM alone was provided ($p <$ 0.01) and to $88.8 \pm 0.8\%$ when HM + H^2MF was provided ($p < 0.05$) (Table 1). Therefore, when the MedFusion™ pump was used, the addition of cream further improved upon the fat delivery efficiency. When the Kangaroo ePump™ was used, an increase in fat delivery efficiency was observed only when both H^2MF and cream were added to HM.

The average total fat (grams) and energy (kcal) delivered by the simulated one-hour feed increased with the addition of H^2MF and further increased with the addition of cream (Table 2).

Table 2. Total fat/calories delivered over 20 mL, one-hour feeds (calculated with right-handed integral approximation).

	HM Fat (g)/Cal (kcal)	HM + H^2MF Fat (g)/Cal (kcal)	HM + H^2MF + cream Fat (g)/Cal (kcal)
Kangaroo ePump™	0.681/12.60	0.873/14.35	1.047/16.04
MedFusion™	0.765/13.55	0.986/16.01	1.178/17.91

HM: human milk; H^2MF: HM supplemented with donor HM-derived fortifier Prolacta + H^2MF™ Cream: HM supplemented with H^2MF and donor HM-derived cream ProlactCR™.

The average fat values at each time point were plotted to show how fat content decreased throughout one-hour simulated feeds (Figures 1 and 2). During simulated feeds using the Kangaroo ePump™, between $t = 0$ to 10 min, the fat content dropped by approximately half of the difference between the fat content at $t = 0$ min and $t = 60$ min (Figure 1). This revealed that a significant proportion of the total fat loss occurred in the first 10 min with all HM variations. By $t = 60$ min, the fat content of HM + H^2MF and HM + H^2MF + cream appeared to stop decreasing, but the fat content of HM continued to decrease after $t = 60$ min due to the negative slope seen in Figure 1. During simulated feeds using the MedFusion™ pump with HM and HM + H^2MF, fat content dropped sharply between $t = 0$ to 5 min and then rose slightly between $t = 5$ to 10 min. After $t = 15$ min, fat levels gradually decreased.

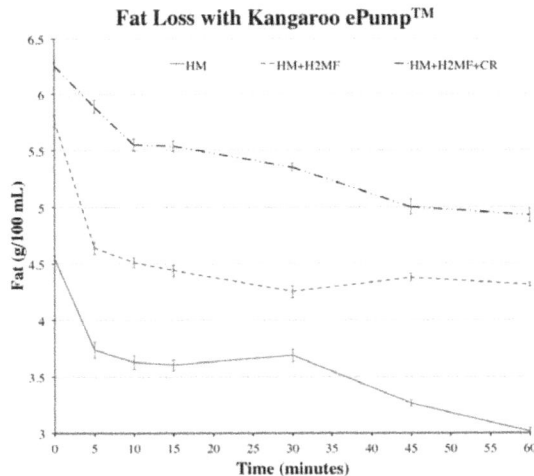

Figure 1. Fat values over one-hour feeds with HM, HM + H^2MF, and HM + H^2MF + cream with Kangaroo ePump™, HM: human milk; H^2MF: HM supplemented with donor HM-derived fortifier Prolacta + H^2MF™; Cream: HM supplemented with H^2MF and donor HM-derived cream ProlactCR™.

Fat Loss with MedFusion™ pump

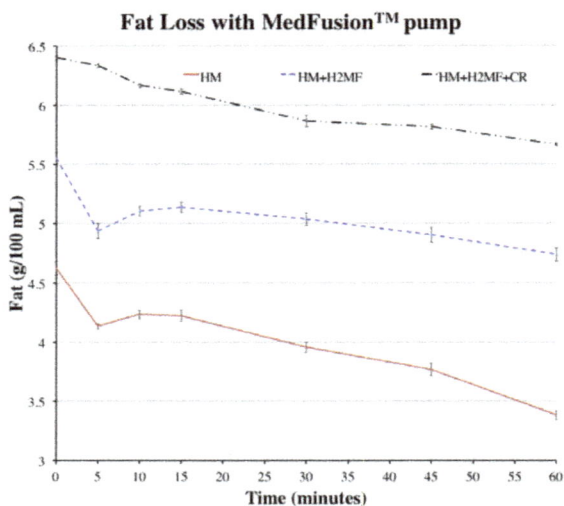

Figure 2. Fat values over one-hour feeds with HM, HM + H^{2}MF, and HM + H^{2}MF + cream with MedFusion™ syringe pump. HM: human milk; H^{2}MF: HM supplemented with donor HM-derived fortifier Prolacta + H^{2}MF™; Cream: HM supplemented with H^{2}MF and donor HM-derived cream ProlactCR™.

Lastly, all data supports the assertion that the MedFusion™ pump resulted in greater fat delivery than the Kangaroo ePump™, in agreement with previous studies. An increase was observed in overall fat delivery efficiency when using the MedFusion™ pump, compared to the Kangaroo ePump™, with each corresponding variation of HM (HM, HM + H^{2}MF, and HM + H^{2}MF + cream) (Table 1). Additionally, the MedFusion™ pump resulted in greater total fat and energy delivered in each variation of HM (Table 2).

4. Discussion

Rogers *et al.* reported that the loss of fat, phosphorus, and calcium during continuous feeding pump methods is substantial, compared to the losses during gravity feeding [5]. Brooks *et al.* also showed a significant increase in fat loss with the MedFusion™ syringe pump compared to gravity feeding [4]. As the amount of fat lost over one-hour feeds is comparable to that lost during two-hour feeds, it appears that most of the fat loss occurs in the first hour.

Few data are available regarding methodologies to decrease fat loss during continuous human milk feedings. Martinez *et al.* results indicate that fat separation can be prevented by ultrasonic homogenization of HM [14]. Furthermore, ultrasonic homogenization of HM appears to improve weight gain and triceps skin-fold thickness in premature neonates by minimizing fat loss, although further testing needs to be done on the safety of this technique [7]. Minibore tubing delivers more fat than standard bore tubing [2], although both types of tubing result in significant fat loss. Increased hydrophilicity of the feeding tube may help minimize clogging [15], and emulsifiers such as carrageenan may increase fat delivery but are currently limited by potential toxicity and lack of practical applicability to human milk feedings [16]. Supplementing enteral nutrition intakes of VLBW infants with H^{2}MF and cream resulted in increased weight gain and length compared to the standard feeding regimen, supporting the use of H^{2}MF and cream as a promising method to promote growth of infants [17].

We evaluated the addition of H^{2}MF and cream as a potential practical method to increase fat delivery with HM. Results suggest that H^{2}MF and cream can be used together to increase the fat delivery efficiency by almost 10% when using the Kangaroo ePump™ or the MedFusion™ syringe pump. The use of H^2MF and cream increases fat delivery while maintaining the benefits of bioactive elements from HM, which may lead to improved weight gain and long-term outcomes.

The calculations in Table 2 can be utilized to approximate the total fat and calories delivered by one-hour feeds at 20 mL·h^{-1} with the corresponding pump type, liquid type, and initial fat content (Figures 1 and 2). The duration of the feed, the flow rate, and the initial fat content of milk affect overall fat delivery efficiency due to fat molecules occupying binding sites on the tubing and bag or syringe. Therefore, in order to accurately predict the total fat and calories delivered by feeds with various conditions, additional experiments must be performed with various feed duration, feed flow rate, and initial fat content. Calculations from these experiments could be utilized to more accurately track the fat that reaches the infant and to plan the appropriate mass of fat delivery in order to achieve proper infant growth rates. Excess fat consumption by infants, as well as insufficient fat consumption, can have negative impacts on childhood health, increasing the importance of tracking fat delivery [18].

Because the addition of H^2MF and cream increases fat delivery efficiency, H^2MF and cream appear to reduce the rate at which fat is lost to the tubing and bag or syringe. H^2MF and cream were formulated through processes involving pasteurization [19], which induces changes in micelles [20], making it possible that H^2MF and cream act as emulsifiers, preventing some of the fat from HM from separating out of the mixture. Alternatively, H^2MF and cream may lose fat at a lower rate than HM loses fat, thereby increasing overall fat delivery efficiency without affecting the fat loss dynamics of HM. Lastly, a combination of these two possibilities may work to increase the overall fat delivery efficiency.

When using the Kangaroo ePump™, significant fat loss in the first 10 minutes of feeds with all HM variations suggests that binding sites on the tubing and bag become saturated more quickly with fat during early stages of the feed. Later in the feed, the rate of fat loss decreases due to the decreased available binding sites. When using HM + H^2MF and HM + H^2MF + cream, which have high initial fat contents, these binding sites fill quickly, causing fat content to approach a lower limit by $t = 60$ min. Different trends of loss occur with the MedFusion™ pump than those with the Kangaroo ePump™, and these differences must be due to the differences between fat loss dynamics in the feeding bag versus the syringe because all other variables were held constant.

Compared to the Kangaroo ePump™, when using the MedFusion™ pump, fat loss in the first 10 min is less rapid, and the overall trend of fat loss appears to be approximately linear. This may occur because the rate of fat molecule separation from the aqueous portion of milk is slower in a horizontal syringe than it is in a vertical feeding bag. The linear trend may be influenced by gradual, continuous fat separation in the syringe coupled with plunger movement. As fat separates toward the plunger end of the syringe, the plunger moves towards the syringe exit, pushing the fat in the same direction. Fat separation may explain the initial sharp drop in fat content, and plunger movement may explain the subsequent slight increase in fat content seen with HM and HM + H^2MF from $t = 5$ to 10 min (Figure 2).

While this study suggests a practical method to increase fat delivery in enteral feeding with HM and provides insight into possible mechanisms of fat loss and retention, it contains the following limitations. Only one flow rate (20 mL·h^{-1}) was tested, and it is known from previous studies that higher flow rates result in greater percent fat retained [7]. All simulated feeds were one hour in duration, but longer feeds will have decreased overall fat delivery efficiencies. Additionally, in a clinical setting, a nasogastric tube is attached to the end of the tubing used in this study, and additional fat loss may occur due to this extra tubing. However, to our knowledge, no studies have quantified the fat lost in nasogastric tubing, and this data can be used as a basis for further investigations designed to evaluate characteristics of fat loss from human milk-based diets.

5. Conclusions

Fat and nutrient loss in continuous enteral feeding methods of HM remains a barrier to providing VLBW infants proper nutrients to grow and survive. Whenever possible, bolus-feeding methods should be utilized in lieu of syringe and pump methods with slow flow rates. However, for those infants who cannot tolerate bolus-feeding, this study proposes the addition of H^2MF and/or cream to HM as a method to increase the percentage of fat delivered during infant enteral feeding. Our results suggests that the addition of H^2MF + cream to HM is a practical method to increase fat delivery to VLBW infants while retaining the benefits of HM, which may lead to increased growth rates and improved long-term outcomes. Exploration of additional solutions to increase fat delivery efficiency at slow flow rates, particularly practical solutions, will provide further benefit for infants requiring enteral nutrition.

Acknowledgments: Baylor College of Medicine, Texas Children's Hospital Milk Bank, Baylor SMART Program.

Author Contributions: M.T. assisted with study design, carried out acquisition and analysis of the data, performed data collection, assisted in interpretation of the data, drafted the manuscript, and approved the final manuscript as submitted.

K.A. carried out acquisition and analysis of the data, performed data collection, assisted in interpretation of the data, drafted the manuscript, and approved the final manuscript as submitted.

A.H. assisted with study design, assisted in interpretation of the data, drafted the manuscript, and approved the final manuscript as submitted.

K.H. assisted with study design, assisted in interpretation of the data, drafted the manuscript, and approved the final manuscript as submitted.

Z.C. assisted with study design and approved the final manuscript as submitted.

S.A. designed the study, supervised interpretation of the data, drafted the manuscript, and approved the final manuscript as submitted.

Conflicts of Interest: ABH received research support from Prolacta Bioscience for the Human Milk Cream Study, which was published in a separate article. She received speaker honoraria from Prolacta Bioscience and Mead Johnson Nutrition. The authors declare no direct conflict of interest. This work is a publication of the U.S. Department of Agriculture (USDA)/Agricultural Research Service (ARS) Children's Nutrition Research Center, Department of Pediatrics, Baylor College of Medicine, and Texas Children's Hospital (Houston, TX, USA). Contents of this publication do not necessarily reflect the views or policies of the USDA, nor does mention of trade names, commercial products, or organizations imply endorsement by the U.S. government.

References

1. Robinson, S.; Fall, C. Infant nutrition and later health: A review of current evidence. *Nutrients* **2012**, *4*, 859–874. [CrossRef] [PubMed]

2. Brennan-Behm, M.; Carlson, G. Caloric loss from expressed mother's milk during continuous gavage infusion. *Neonatal. Netw.* **1994**, *13*, 27–32. [PubMed]

3. Brooke, O.; Barley, J. Loss of energy during continuous infusions of breast milk. *Arch. Dis. Child* **1978**, *53*, 344–345. [CrossRef] [PubMed]

4. Brooks, C.; Vickers, A.M.; Aryal, S. Comparison of lipid and calorie loss from donor human milk among 3 methods of simulated gavage feeding. *Adv. in Neon. Care.* **2013**, *13*, 131–138.

5. Rogers, S.P.; Hicks, P.D.; Hamzo, M.; Veit, L.E.; Abrams, S.A. Continuous feedings of fortified human milk lead to nutrient losses of fat, calcium and phosphorus. *Nutrients* **2010**, *2*, 230–240.

6. Stocks, R.; Davies, D.; Allen, F.; Sewell, D. Loss of breast milk nutrients during tube feeding. *Arch. Dis. Child.* **1985**, *60*, 164–166.

7. Rayol, M.; Martinez, F.; Jorge, S. Feeding premature infants banked human milk homogenized by ultrasonic treatment. *J. Pediatr.* **1993**, *123*, 985–988. [CrossRef] [PubMed]

8. Sullivan, S.; Schanler, R.J.; Kim, J.H.; Patel, A.L.; Trawöger, R.; Kiechl-Kohlendorfer, U.; Chan, G.M.; Blanco, C.L.; Cotton, C.M.; *et al.* An exclusively human milk-based diet is associated with a lower rate of necrotizing enterocolitis than a diet of human milk and bovine milk-based products. *J. Pediatr.* **2010**, *156*, 562–567.

9. Cristofalo, E.A.; Schanler, R.J.; Blanco, C.L.; Sullivan, S.; Trawoeger, R.; Kiechl-Kohlendorfer, U.; Dudell, G.; Rechtman, D.J.; Lee, M.L.; Lucas, A.; *et al.* Randomized trial of exclusive human milk versus preterm formula diets in extremely premature infants. *J. Pediatr.* **2013**, *163*, 1592–1595.

10. Abrams, S.A.; Schanler, R.J.; Lee, M.L.; Rechtman, D.J.; the H^2MF Study Group. Greater mortality and morbidity in extremely preterm infants fed a diet containing cow milk protein products. *Breastfeeding Med.* **2014**, *9*, 281–285.

11. Product Literature. Available online: http://www.prolacta.com/data/sites/14/media/products/MKT-0264Rev-1ProlactCR_SPI.pdf (accessed on 16 January 2014).

12. Halleux, V.D.; Rigo, J. Variability in human milk composition: Benefit of individualized fortification in very-low birth-weight infants. *Am. J. Clin. Nutr.* **2013**, *98*, 529–535. [CrossRef]

13. Fusch, G.; Rochow, N.; Choi, A.; Fusch, S.; Poeschl, S.; Ubah, A.; Lee, O.; Raja, S.Y.; Fusch, P. Rapid measurement of macronutrients in breast milk: How reliable are infrared milk analyzers? *Clin. Nutr.* **2014**, in press.

14. Martinez, F.; Desai, I.; Davidson, A. Ultrasonic homogenization of expressed human milk to prevent fat loss during tube feeding. *J. Pediatr. Gastroenterol. Nutr.* **1987**, *6*, 593–597. [CrossRef] [PubMed]

15. Gaither, K.A.; Tarasevich, B.J.; Goheen, S.C. Modification of polyurethane to reduce occlusion of enteral feeding tubes. *J. Biomed. Mater. Res. B Appl. Biomater.* **2009**, *91*, 135–142. [CrossRef] [PubMed]

16. Weiner, M.L. Toxicological properties of carrageenan. *Agents Actions* **1991**, *32*, 46–51. [CrossRef] [PubMed]

17. Hair, A.B.; Blanco, C.L.; Moreira, A.G.; Hawthorne, K.M.; Lee, M.L.; Rechtman, D.J.; Abrams, S.A. Randomized trial of human milk cream as a supplement to standard fortification of an exclusive human milk-based diet in infants 750–1250 g birth weight. *J. Pediatr.* **2014**, *5*, 915–920. [CrossRef]

18. Stettler, N.; Zemel, B.S.; Kumanyika, S.; Stallings, V.A. Infant weight gain and childhood overweight status in multicenter, cohort study. *Pediatrics* **2002**, *109*, 194–199. [CrossRef] [PubMed]

19. Product Literature. Available online: http://www.prolacta.com/why-the-need-for-fortification-1 (accessed on 16 November 2014).

20. Huppertz, T.; Kelly, A.L.; Fox, P.F. Effects of high pressure on constituents and properties of milk. *Int. Dairy J.* **2002**, *12*, 561–572. [CrossRef]

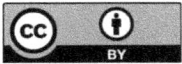

nutrients

MDPI

Article

Development and Evaluation of a Home Enteral Nutrition Team

Sarah Dinenage [1], Morwenna Gower [2], Joanna Van Wyk [3], Anne Blamey [1], Karen Ashbolt [1], Michelle Sutcliffe [1] and Sue M. Green [4,*]

[1] University Hospital Southampton NHS Foundation Trust, Southampton, Hampshire, SO16 6YD, UK; sarah.dinenage@nhs.net (S.D.); anne.blamey@uhs.nhs.uk (A.B.); Karen.ashbolt@uhs.nhs.uk (K.A.); michelle.sutcliffe@nhs.net (M.S.)
[2] Solent NHS Trust, Adelaide Health Centre, Western Community Hospital Campus, Southampton, SO16 4XE, UK; morwenna.gower@solent.nhs.uk
[3] Nutricia Ltd., Trowbridge, Wiltshire, BA14 0XQ, UK; Johanna.vanwyk@nutricia.com
[4] Solent NHS Trust/University of Southampton, Highfield, Southampton, SO17 1BJ, UK
* Author to whom correspondence should be addressed; S.M.Green@soton.ac.uk.

Received: 3 December 2014; Accepted: 12 February 2015; Published: 5 March 2015

Abstract: The organisation of services to support the increasing number of people receiving enteral tube feeding (ETF) at home varies across regions. There is evidence that multi-disciplinary primary care teams focussed on home enteral nutrition (HEN) can provide cost-effective care. This paper describes the development and evaluation of a HEN Team in one UK city. A HEN Team comprising dietetians, nurses and a speech and language therapist was developed with the aim of delivering a quality service for people with gastrostomy tubes living at home. Team objectives were set and an underpinning framework of organisation developed including a care pathway and a schedule of training. Impact on patient outcomes was assessed in a pre-post test evaluation design. Patients and carers reported improved support in managing their ETF. Cost savings were realised through: (1) prevention of hospital admission and related transport for ETF related issues; (2) effective management and reduction of waste of feed and thickener; (3) balloon gastrostomy tube replacement by the HEN Team in the patient's home, and optimisation of nutritional status. This service evaluation demonstrated that the establishment of a dedicated multi-professional HEN Team focussed on achievement of key objectives improved patient experience and, although calculation of cost savings were estimates, provided evidence of cost-effectiveness.

Keywords: Enteral tube feeding; home enteral nutrition; primary care

1. Introduction

The number of people receiving food and fluid intake via a gastrostomy tube in primary care has increased [1,2] and it is now a relatively common intervention in the UK [3]. Poorly managed gastrostomy tubes and enteral feeding in the community setting can lead to complications, hospital admission [3] and dissatisfaction with care provision [4]. Other aspects of poor management include wastage of feeds and equipment. Therefore, it is important that people with gastrostomy tubes, their carers and primary care services are supported to manage the therapy effectively.

Management of a gastrostomy tube at home requires development of knowledge and skills and life style adaptations. People with a gastrostomy tube report it to be a burden, time-consuming and disruptive to their lives [5,6]. Further, relatives of people living at home with a feeding tube have described managing the new life situation it presents as a struggle [4]. Appropriate education, training and support is required both to ensure a smooth transition between care settings and safe and effective management within the primary care setting [7,8]. UK NICE guidelines [9] outline that people receiving enteral tube feeding (ETF) in the community should "be supported by a coordinated multidisciplinary team". There are a number of ways services can be organised to support people with home enteral feeding (HEF) [10] and a range of intervention strategies have been described [11]. A recent systematic review highlighted that a standardised care coordination model with a multidisciplinary team can improve patient outcomes and reduce health care costs, but there is insufficient evidence to determine the effectiveness of a particular intervention or team composition [11]. Outpatient-based services, such as enteral nutrition support clinics, have been suggested to improve care quality and reduce hospital readmissions, tube-related complications and costs [12]. In some areas, teams based in community settings (often termed Home Enteral Nutrition (HEN) teams) have been formed to provide a service for patients in their own homes [13] and these have been associated with improved care outcomes. For example, Klek *et al.* [14] report cost savings following the introduction of commercial formulas and guidance from a nutrition support team. In the UK, Kurian *et al.* [3] suggested that the direct actions of a HEN Team comprising dietitians and assistants in one UK city potentially resulted in the avoidance of 227 hospital admissions over a year. This paper aims to describe the development, interventions and evaluation of a multidisplinary HEN Team in one city in England.

2. Materials and Methods

2.1. Team Development

Local funding was secured for six months to form a HEN Team and scope the potential for improved patient care and cost savings. Following this, a further 12 months of funding totaling £84,071 was awarded, which allowed the service to be embedded in local healthcare provision. The Team comprised a dietitian, a speech and language therapist, a homecare company nurse and a nutrition nurse. All Team members worked part-time with the Team whilst holding other professional roles within their contracted time.

2.2. Team Aim and Objectives

The aim of the HEN Team was to provide a service for people over the age of 18 with gastrostomy tubes in a UK city (population approximately 265,000) focussed on improving patient experience and quality of nutritional care. The key objectives for the Team and how they were achieved are outlined below to give information on the interventions and how they were implemented.

2.2.1. Objective: Development of a Care Pathway and Links with Other Services

An integrated care pathway in the form of a flow chart was developed and embedded into practice (Figure 1). The pathway outlined the stages of management for people concerning their feeding tubes, including how referrals were created, timeframes for assessment and review, and discharge from the service. The roles and responsibilities of each Team member were also outlined. The pathway provided a framework for activity and acted as a point of reference. Communication with other teams (such as the acute dietetic service and the local Nutrition Support Team) involved in caring for people with enteral feeding tubes enabled the development of professional networks which facilitated and improved coordination of care.

2.2.2. Objective: Care Provision with Reference to NICE Guidelines [8,9]

The Team provided a service delivering multidisciplinary care concerning nutrition for adults with gastrostomy tubes in the home setting. The following activities were undertaken with each patient:

- Review of use of feed ancillaries (giving sets, syringes, connectors, replacement parts), feed, thickener prescription and adjustment of plan of care if required on admission to the service and at least 6 monthly subsequently
- Review of stoma and tube and adjustment of plan of care if required
- Repair of tube as required
- Planned and emergency balloon-retained gastrostomy tube replacement at home where not clinically contraindicated
- Review of type of balloon-retained gastrostomy tubes and change to longer-lasting tubes requiring fewer balloon volume checks where possible
- Review of route and preparation of medication and suggestions for change if appropriate

An individualised care plan for gastrostomy and nutritional management was developed for each patient. As well as providing support for patients and carers, the Team worked to reduce risks through the early identification of problems.

2.2.3. Objective: Provision of Specialist Advice, Training and Education

The Team acted as a source of specialist advice on home ETF for patients, carers and other community practitioners. Members of the Team could be contacted by telephone during office hours. The Homecare Company continued to provide a 24 h helpline as part of their service contract. Relevant training and education was delivered to patients, carers, family members and nursing home staff in the form of in-house training and a study day.

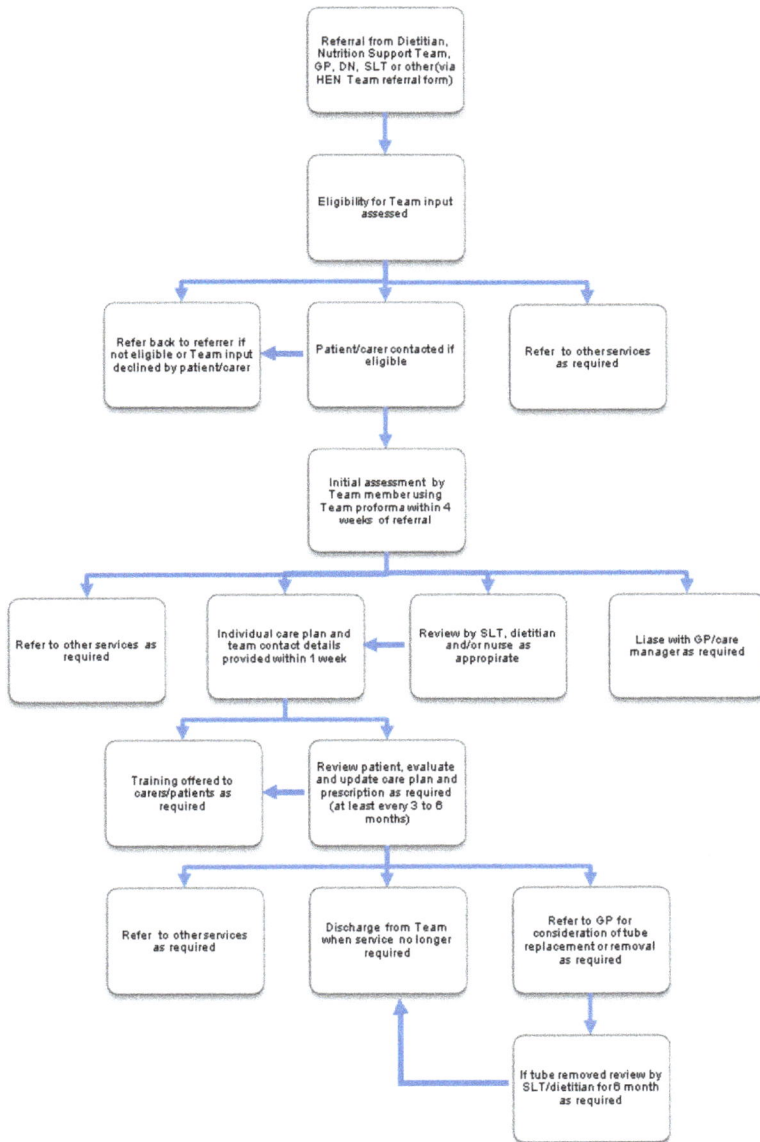

Figure 1. Care pathway for management of patients with enteral tubes by Home Enteral Nutrition (HEN) Team, Key: GP: General practitioner, DN: district nurse, SLT: Speech and language therapist.

2.2.4. Service Evaluation

A pre-post evaluation of the impact of the presence of the HEN Team on selected patient outcomes derived from the HEN Team objectives outlined above was undertaken. Outcomes (except those related to hospital admission) for all 70 patients in the caseload were compared at one time point in the 12 months pre-HEN Team development (2011) and one time point following the first three months of the Team development (2012) or at the point of discharge from the Team. From this, the mean cost per day for each patient was calculated.

Hospital admission costs were calculated for 28 patients. This convenience sample was selected on the basis of known hospital admission. Sample size was determined by the time available to extract data from the hospital medical records recorded over a 24-month period. For these 28 patients, the mean cost per year of hospital admission was calculated from the review of 24 months of medical records pre-HEN Team development. These were then compared with the mean cost for 2012.

2.2.5. Outcomes Included

- Number of patients whose risk of malnutrition decreased (measured using the Malnutrition Universal Screening Tool (MUST) [15])
- Number of patients, carers, healthcare staff and nursing home trained in gastrostomy tube care
- Number of patients who had tubes removed
- Estimates of cost of:

  ○ enteral feed prescription
  ○ thickening agents for dysphagia

- Frequency and length of hospital admission and hospital transport costs for ETF related problems for 28 patients in the caseload.

Data was obtained from hospital medical, dietetic, and community and homecare nursing records. A patient satisfaction survey in the form of a written questionnaire was undertaken at one time point during the 12 months. The survey comprised a 15-item anonymous postal questionnaire which was adapted from an existing service evaluation. The two items reported here concern the questions "Before your first appointment, did you know what to expect from the HEN Team?" (yes or no) and "How they would you rate the overall service received? (very poor, poor, OK, good or excellent).

This was distributed to all patients in the caseload by post with a stamped addressed envelope for return.

2.3. Statistical Analysis

SPSS 17.0 was used to record and analyse data using descriptive statistics and frequencies. Actual cost savings were estimated. Values for bed days were calculated using the following estimates derived from service managers and a Trust Finance Department: day case £250, general medical ward £177, acute medical unit (AMU) £240, critical care £1100, specialist rehabilitation unit £470. If the admission location was unclear, costs were calculated as 2 days on AMU and the remainder on a general medical ward. The cost of patient transport relating to hospital admissions was calculated using an average price of £55.77 per trip. The cost of feed and thickener for each patient per day was calculated and then an estimated cost per year obtained for each patient. These were then summed to produce an annual cost. Products were costed using the invoice supplied by the provider or from the current British National Formulary. Costs of gastrostomy tubes were obtained from manufacturers. Scheduled time in the radiology department was estimated at £250 per case.

2.4. Ethics and Governance

The study was registered as a service evaluation with the Trust and deemed not to require ethical committee approval. Confidentiality was maintained during the recording and analysis of the data. Personal identifying information was not recorded and patients were allocated a unique anonymous identification number.

3. Results

3.1. Caseload Characteristics

People from the age of 18 years and older were admitted to the caseload, although the mean age was 61 years (range 19 to 90 years). The majority of patients were female (60%). Nearly 70% lived in their own homes with the remainder living in nursing homes. A high proportion of patients (approximately 70%) had a percutaneously inserted gastrostomy tube. The remainder had a balloon retained gastrostomy (about 20%), "low-profile" gastrostomy or jejunostomy. The most frequently reported medical condition causing the need for a tube was cerebrovascular accident (about 25%) but other conditions that featured frequently in the population were neurological diseases and learning disability [16].

The HEN Team made a total of 595 contacts (face to face and via telephone) over the course of 2012, equating to a mean of 50 contacts per month or 8.5 contacts per patient over the year. A breakdown of contacts per discipline is shown in Table 1.

Table 1. Contacts by discipline.

	Dietitian	Speech and Language Therapist	Nurse	TOTAL
Number of contacts	241	187	167	595

3.2. Must Score

The proportion of patients at medium or high risk of malnutrition (MUST score greater than 0) was reduced from 41% to 25% suggesting reduced risk of malnutrition.

3.3. Training

Each patient, and where appropriate their carers, received training at the point of care. A study day entitled "Caring for tube feeds in the community" was held by the HEN Team and attended by 20 healthcare professionals and carers during the intervention period. The study day was not available in the pre-intervention period.

3.4. Number of Patients Who Had Tubes Removed

Over the course of the intervention period (2012) eight patients had their tubes removed, which is broadly in line with other published reports [3].

3.5. Estimated Cost Savings

Table 2 shows estimates of the cost savings for specific components of the care provision pre and post intervention.

Review of each patient's enteral feed prescription by the dietitian, to ensure patient nutritional needs were being met, resulted in cost savings because some feeds were reduced or changed to standard feeds and bolus feeds (Table 2). Review of water and feed ancillaries for each patient resulted in some adjustments made to their equipment supply to ensure unnecessary components were not ordered and supplies were not excessive. For example, one patient was initially receiving two 500 mL bags of a concentrated feed with a two-pack connector. Following dietetic assessment, the patient was changed over to one bag of a high-energy feed, thus removing the need for the two-pack connector as well as reducing the number of bags of feed. This prescription was more appropriate for the patient as it was less labour-intensive. The cost savings as a result of review of water and feed ancillaries are not included in the calucation of the cost savings.

Table 2. Estimated costs pre and post introduction of the Home Enteral Nutrition Team (*n* = 70).

Component of provision	Calculation of estimated costs	Pre introduction estimated cost (2011)	Post introduction estimated cost (2012)	Estimated Cost differential
Enteral feed prescription per year	2011: mean cost of feed £9.18 per patient per day 2012: mean cost of feed £7.41 per patient per day	£234,505	£189,326	£45,179
Thickening agents for dysphagia	2011: daily thickener costs per patient £0.53 2012: daily thickener costs per patient £0.48	£13,542	£12,264	£1,278

Review of thickening agent use and type by the speech and language therapist resulted in cost savings as swallow ability of some patients improved (Table 2).

There were fewer hospital admissions for tube-related problems recorded in 2012 compared to 2010/2011 (Table 3). There were also fewer hospital admissions for routine balloon gastrostomy tube replacement. Over the course of 2012, the Team undertook tube replacement in the home for fourteen patients. Prior to the introduction of the HEN Team, some patients were attending radiology to have their balloon gastrostomy tube replaced. Manufacturers guidelines for the type of tube routinely used within the local area suggest three monthly replacements, so this potentially saved four radiology appointments yearly per patient. Additionally, over the course of 2012, seven patients were changed to a tube type which requires checking of the balloon volume and changing less frequently than the previous tube routinely used. This resulted in a reduction in tube cost of £93 per patient or £651 for the year. Cost of nurse visits to change the balloon volume were not calculated.

3.6. Patient Satisfaction Survey

Fourteen people returned the patient satisfaction survey (30% response rate). All respondents stated that they were were extremely satisfied with the services provided by the HEN Team, with 100% of respondents rating the overall service received as good or excellent. Over half the respondents to the survey indicated that they had not known what to expect from the HEN Team before the first visit, suggesting that the role of the HEN Team was unclear.

Table 3. Estimated costs of hospital admission pre and post introduction of the Home Enteral Nutrition Team (*n* = 28).

Costs component	Calculation of estimated saving	Pre-introduction estimated cost (mean per year)	Post-introduction estimated cost (2012)	Estimated cost differential
Hospital admission (frequency and bed days) for balloon gastrostomy tube replacement and tube related problems	2010/2011: • 25 admissions • 740 bed days • 10 day cases 2012: • 7 admissions • 98 bed days • 2 day cases	£82,943	£18,602	£64,341
Hospital transport for balloon gastrostomy tube replacement in hospital and tube related problems	2010/2011: Transport based on 25 admissions and 10 day cases 2012: Transport based on 7 hospital admissions and 2 day cases	£976	£502	£474

Nutrients **2015**, *7*, 1607–1617

4. Discussion

Increasingly, community services are required to support people with ETF [17]. It is important to consider how a service can be provided that effectively meets the needs of patients, as currently there is little guidance on who should be included in the Team, the implementation process or evaluation of effectiveness [11]. The introduction of a new team to deliver a service previously not available in the local area was approached by forming team aims and objectives linked with clear measurable outcomes. This enabled care provision concerning ETF via gastrostomy to align closely with national guidelines [8,9] and expected standards of care [18]. The service evaluation measured by the outcomes generated from the team objectives indicated that the Team was able to provide a cost-effective community service, which improved the experience and quality of care of people with gastrostomy tubes. For a cohort of 70 patients, the introduction of a HEN Team was associated with crude estimated cost savings of £111,272 over one year. The service cost £84,071 to deliver, giving rise to an estimated net saving of £27,201 to the NHS.

Previous evaluations of similar teams have demonstrated greater cost savings [3]. Other activities of the HEN Team linked to the Team objectives potentially generated further costs savings but were not included in the cost savings analysis presented in this paper. These included review of ancillaries and water ordered for each patient, review of medications and transfer to oral medication with improved swallow, reduction in dressing use as a result of improved training, reduction in district nursing time for balloon volume changes, and recommendation for removal of gastrostomy tubes where swallow function improved sufficiently to enable adequate oral intake to maintain health. Calculating cost savings was a challenge for the Team, as it was an activity that none of the members had previously undertaken. The estimates of savings were crude, being based on figures that were estimates of cost. Nevertheless, some cost savings were clearly made. Other reported evaluations of teams have focussed on measurement of patient-reported outcome measures to demonstrate clinical effectiveness [19]; however, we considered it essential to demonstrate cost effectiveness in addition to patient satisfaction. A recent systematic review identified that evaluation of cost effectiveness of nursing practice is limited [20] and there is a need to consider cost implications in service delivery within community settings.

The multidisciplinary nature of the Team enabled rapid referral to other disciplines, consistent advice, more regular review, timely and appropriate clinical care and better provision of training. The speech and language therapist was a key member of the Team. She supported and empowered patients with dysphagia to comply with clinical recommendations concerning food and fluid intake. In addition, as each patient's ability to swallow was reviewed regularly, any patient with the potential for improved swallow received ongoing speech and language therapy at home. This potentially reduced the risk of aspiration pneumonia and, for some patients, resulted in timely removal of their gastrostomy tube. This has a significant impact on patient experience. The psychosocial benefits of receiving oral intake should not be underestimated.

4.1. Limitations

The time since insertion of the tube was not taken into account in calculation of the cost savings. This is a limitation of this study as it has been suggested that there is a substantial risk of complications in the first few months of placement [21]. A design that allowed for a control group would have been preferable but was not feasible as a result of service requirements. Calculated cost savings were crude estimates due to the clinical Team's inexperience in undertaking robust economic evaluation. However, it was considered important to attempt to demonstrate the value for the service to the local NHS economy, and demonstrates the need for clinicians to develop skills in evaluation of cost effectiveness of services. The pre-post intervention evaluation design did not allow for temporal variations in care environment to be evaluated, and the changes seen may have occurred without the introduction of the Team.

Nutrients **2015**, *7*, 1607–1617

4.2. Practice Recommendations

A HEN Team has the potential to increase patient satisfaction and reduce costs associated with ETF in the community. The process of team development requires the setting of clear aims and key objectives focussed on enhancing patient experience. When implementing a specialist community healthcare service, it is important to consider how the service can be evaluated robustly so patient satisfaction and cost-effectiveness can be demonstrated.

5. Conclusion

ETF is a costly therapy, and a dedicated HEN Team can help to minimise the significant costs related to tube feeding and enhance the experience of people receiving tube feeding at home. These findings are consistent with other similar studies [11]. Through effective management and care delivery, it was shown that patients supported by the HEN Team were admitted to hospital less frequently, used less hospital transport and had reduced costs for feed and thickener. The reduction in hospital admissions is likely to be due to risk management by the HEN Team for complications such as tube blockage and deterioration. However, as the study design was pre- and post-evaluation, hospital admission may have been reduced as a function of time. Other components of the provision not measured would have been likely to contribute to costs savings.

Acknowledgments: The authors would like to acknowledge Hilary Warwick for her part in the development of the Team and advice on outcomes.

Author Contributions: AB and MS were involved in the conception of the Team. All authors were involved in the development of the Team and service evaluation. SD and MG analysed the data and calculated the costs savings. SG, SD and MG wrote the paper for submission.

Conflicts of Interest: Johanna Van Wuck is employed by Nutricia Homeward which provides a home enteral nutrition service. No other conflicts of interest are declared.

References

1. Russell, C.A.; Rollins, H. The needs of patients requiring home enteral tube feeding. *Prof. Nurs.* **2002**, *17*, 500–502.
2. British Association of Enteral and Parenteral Nutrition. *Annual BANS Report*; Smith, T., Ed.; The British Association for Parenteral and Enteral Nutrition: Redditch, UK, 2011; pp. 1–50. Available online: http://www.bapen.org.ukn (accessed on 18 February 2015).
3. Kurien, M.; White, S.; Simpson, G.; Grant, J.; Sanders, D.S.; McAlindon, M.E. Managing patients with gastrostomy tubes in the community: Can a dedicated enteral feed dietetic service reduce hospital readmissions? *Eur. J. Clin. Nutr.* **2012**, *66*, 757–760. [CrossRef] [PubMed]
4. Bjuresäter, K.; Larsson, M.; Athlin, E. Struggling in an inescapable life situation: Being a close relative of a person dependent on home enteral tube feeding. *J. Clin. Nurs.* **2012**, *21*, 1051–1059. [CrossRef] [PubMed]
5. Jordan, S.; Philpin, S.; Warring, J.; Cheung, W.Y.; Williams, J. Percutaneous endoscopic gastrostomies: the burden of treatment from a patient perspective. *J. Adv. Nurs.* **2006**, *56*, 270–281. [CrossRef] [PubMed]
6. Martin, L.; Blomberg, J.; Lagergren, P. Patients' perspectives of living with a percutaneous endoscopic gastrostomy (PEG). *BMC Gastroenterol.* **2012**, *12*, 126. [CrossRef] [PubMed]
7. National Institute for Health and Clinical Excellence. *Infection: Prevention and control of healthcare-associated infections in primary and community care*; NICE: London, UK, 2012; pp. 1–47.
8. National Institute for Health and Clinical Excellence. *Quality standard for nutrition support in adults*; NICE: Manchester, UK, 2012; pp. 1–33.
9. National Institute for Health and Clinical Excellence. *Nutritional Support in Adults: Oral Nutrition Support, Enteral Tube Feeding*; NICE: London, UK, 2006; pp. 1–49.
10. Green, S.; Dinenage, S.; Gower, M.; Van Wyk, J. Home enteral nutrition: Organisation of services. *Nurs. Older People* **2013**, *25*, 14–18. [CrossRef] [PubMed]

11. Majka, A.J.; Wang, Z.; Schmitz, K.R.; Niesen, C.R.; Larsen, R.A.; Kinsey, G.C.; Murad, A.L.; Prokop, L.J.; Murad, M.H. Care coordination to enhance management of long-term enteral tube feeding: A systematic review and meta-analysis. *J. Parenter. Enter. Nutr.* **2014**, *38*, 40–52. [CrossRef]

12. Hall, B.T.; Englehart, M.S.; Blaseg, K.; Wessel, K.; Stawicki, S.P.; Evans, D.C. Implementation of a dietitian-led enteral nutrition support clinic results in quality improvement, reduced readmissions, and cost savings. *Nutr. Clin. Prac.* **2014**, *29*, 649–655. [CrossRef]

13. Omorogieva, O.; Patel, I. Home enteral nutrition and team working. *J. Community Nurs.* **2012**, *26*, 15–18.

14. Klek, S.; Szybinski, P.; Sierzega, M.; Szczepanek, K.; Sumlet, M.; Kupiec, M.; Koczur-Szozda, E.; Steinhoff-Nowak, M.; Figula, K.; Kowalczyk, T.; *et al.* Commercial enteral formulas and nutrition support teams improve the outcome of home enteral tube feeding. *JPEN* **2011**, *35*, 380–385. [CrossRef]

15. British Association for Parenteral and Enteral Nutrition. Introducing "MUST". Available online: http://www.bapen.org.uk/screening-for-malnutrition/must/introducing-must (accessed on 18 February 2015).

16. Department of Health. Valuing People: A New Strategy for Learning Disability for the 21st Century. Department of Health: London, UK, 2001; pp. 1–142.

17. McLaughlin, K.A. Home sweet home-can future enteral tube feeding for motor neurone disease begin in the community. *CN* **2014**, *14*, 35–37.

18. Care Quality Commission. Essential Standards of Quality and Safety. Care Quality Commission: London, UK, 2010; pp. 1–278.

19. Bermange, J.; Stewart, K. Measuring clinical outcomes in a community home enteral feeding team. *CN* **2013**, *13*, 50–52.

20. Lämås, K.; Willman, A.; Lindholm, L.; Jacobsson, C. Economic evaluation of nursing practices: A review of literature. *Int. Nurs. Rev.* **2009**, *56*, 13–20. [CrossRef] [PubMed]

21. Blomberg, J.; Lagergren, J.; Martin, L.; Mattsson, F.; Lagergren, P. Complications after percutaneous endoscopic gastrostomy in a prospective study. *Scan. J. Gastroenterol.* **2012**, *47*, 737–742. [CrossRef]

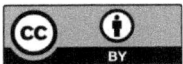

nutrients

MDPI

Review

Enteral Nutrition Support to Treat Malnutrition in Inflammatory Bowel Disease

Roberta Altomare [1,†], **Giuseppe Damiano** [2,†], **Alida Abruzzo** [1], **Vincenzo Davide Palumbo** [1], **Giovanni Tomasello** [2,3], **Salvatore Buscemi** [1] and **Attilio Ignazio Lo Monte** [2,3,*]

[1] School in Surgical Biotechnology and Regenerative Medicine, School of Medicine, School of Biotechnology, University of Palermo, Via del Vespro 129, Palermo 90127, Italy; roberta.altomare@unipa.it (R.A.); alida.abruzzo@unipa.it (A.A.); vincenzodavide.palumbo@unipa.it (V.D.P.); salvatore.buscemi@unipa.it (S.B.)
[2] AUOP "P.Giaccone", Universitary Hospital, Via del Vespro 129, Palermo 90127, Italy; guise.damiano@gmail.com (G.D.); giovanni.tomasello@unipa.it (G.T.)
[3] GENURTO Department, School of Medicine and Biotechnology, University of Palermo, Via del Vespro 129, Palermo 90127, Italy
[*] Author to whom correspondence should be addressed; attilioignazio.lomonte@unipa.it; Tel.: +39-091-655-37-43; Fax: +39-091-655-26-63.
[†] These authors contributed equally to this work.

Received: 15 December 2014; Accepted: 6 January 2015; Published: 25 March 2015

Abstract: Malnutrition is a common consequence of inflammatory bowel disease (IBD). Diet has an important role in the management of IBD, as it prevents and corrects malnutrition. It is well known that diet may be implicated in the aetiology of IBD and that it plays a central role in the pathogenesis of gastrointestinal-tract disease. Often oral nutrition alone is not sufficient in the management of IBD patients, especially in children or the elderly, and must be combined with oral supplementation or replaced with tube enteral nutrition. In this review, we describe several different approaches to enteral nutrition—total parenteral, oral supplementation and enteral tube feeding—in terms of results, patients compliance, risks and and benefits. We also focus on the home entaral nutrition strategy as the future goal for treating IBD while focusing on patient wellness.

Keywords: enteral feeding; malnutrition; nutrients supplementation; inflammatory bowel disease; tube feeding; home enteral nutrition

1. Introduction

Enteral nutritional therapy aims to maintain or restore the nutritional status of individuals who fail to maintain a sufficient oral intake, despite having a fully or partially functioning gastrointestinal tract. Its administration is related to the reduction of infectious complications and maintenance of the integrity of intestinal flora [1]. Lesions of the jaw and central nervous system, anorexia, cancer, hypermetabolic conditions such as burns and severe infections, and, above all, IBD are examples for enteral nutrition indicators [1,2].

The term IBD includes at least three clinical conditions: ulcerative colitis (UC), Crohn's disease (CD) and indeterminate colitis (IC). IBD can occur at all ages and in both genders. Patients usually complain of severe diarrhea, abdominal pain, weight loss and fever, which severely interfere with their quality of life. Understanding the aetiology of IBD is still controversial as it is a multifactorial pathology; it likely depends on an interaction between susceptible genes and environmental factors leading to an abnormal chronic immunological response that causes tissue injury with bowel inflammation and ulceration [2,3].

It is known that the diet plays a role in the pathogenesis of IBD, as has been demonstrated by exclusion diets in several studies [4]. However, it is possible that some nutrients act either as antigens or have therapeutic effects in the intestinal mucosa [2].

In both UC and CD, nutritional deficiencies of various severities are often found. These include protein-energy malnutrition and various vitamin, mineral and trace element deficiencies [5]. Malnutrition in IBD depends on several factors such as inflammatory processes, impaired intestinal absorption, nutrients loss through the inflamed and ulcerated gut, bacterial overgrowth, medical management with steroids or imposed dietary restrictions [2,5].

These observations suggest that nutritional support may be the best approach to treat IBD instead of using drugs, as it could control inflammation and treat malnutrition without side effects.

The first attempt to use enteral nutrition as primary therapy in IBD was made with amino acid-based elemental diets in patients with active CD. The concept was that providing amino acids (elemental diets) instead of intact proteins (polymeric diets) would decrease the intestinal antigenic load in the gut lumen, which in turn would decrease the chances of triggering or maintaining the abnormal or up-regulated inflammatory bowel response. Elemental diets have been shown to decrease intestinal permeability and diminish the excretion of pro-inflammatory cytokines in the stools in CD patients [6,7].

One of the most important goals of nutritional therapy should be to prevent and treat undernutrition, improving the growth and development of children and adolescents using total parenteral nutrition (TPN), enteral nutrition (EN), or by correcting micronutrient deficiency [8,9].

2. Feeding Methods and Patients Management

Sip feeding, tube feeding and parenteral nutrition have all been tested and found to be comparably effective. The selection of the form of nutritional therapy is therefore dependent on secondary factors such as cost, side effects and inconvenience for the patient. Based on these considerations, enteral tube feeding is the primary choice for nutritional therapy of an active phase of Crohn's disease. The mechanism by which nutritional therapy affects the active phase of Crohn's disease is not clear. Two hypotheses have been discussed: (1) bowel rest with reduction of luminal bacteria and antigens leading to a decrease in inflammation; and (2) induction of anabolism changing the immune reaction and thereby reducing inflammation. It is likely that both mechanisms contribute.

Tube feeding is the preferred nutritional therapy for the active phase of Crohn's disease. Sip feeding is similarly effective, provided that patients drink enough from the diet to meet their requirements. This is difficult to achieve, however. Sip feeding is hampered by a high rate of non-compliance due to the poor palatability of the diets. Therefore, until more palatable diets are available, patients should be offered tube feeding as the treatment of first choice [10].

2.1. Total Parenteral Nutrition (TPN)

TPN, although it is the only way of putting the bowel at complete rest, has not been shown to be superior to tube feeding. It may be indicated in some restricted cases, such as in an obstructed bowel that is not amenable to feeding tube placement beyond the obstruction, a short bowel resulting in severe malabsorption or fluid and electrolyte loss that cannot be managed enterally, severe dysmotility in which enteral feeding is impossible, a leaking intestine from high-output intestinal fistula or surgical anastomotic breakdown, in patients intolerant to EN whose feeding cannot be maintained orally, when there is an inability to access the gut for enteral feeding, and in patients undergoing IBD-related bowel surgery in the perioperative period [8,11].

Available data so far show that while artificial nutrition seems to play a primary role in the management of patients with active CD, it does not have a primary therapeutic effect in active UC and does not induce clinical remission of this type of IBD [12].

The use of TPN in the management of active CD is based on theoretical advantages including bowel rest, which could reduce the motor and transport functions of the diseased bowel; reduction of antigenic stimulation, which could eliminate the immunological response to food favored by the presence of impaired intestinal permeability; and stimulation of protein synthesis, which could lead to cell renewal and mucosal healing in the intestine [13]. Nevertheless, few controlled clinical trials have been conducted on the use of TPN to induce remission in active CD. The remission rate three months after starting TPN varied from 20% to 79%, depending on the patient population, length of TPN administration, definitions of remission or recurrence, and concomitant use of medication [14]. TPN has also been shown to achieve fistula healing in 43–63% of patients, accompanied by disease activity reduction and weight gain [15]. TPN was also associated with an increased risk of adverse events such as sepsis and cholestatic liver disease [12].

2.2. Enteral Nutrition (EN)

In addition to the fact that it delivers normal food, EN (with oral nutritional supplements or tube feeding) may be more useful than TPN in the management of undernourished patients with IBD. If the gut can be used safely, EN is actually the preferred feeding method for CD or UC patients who need nutritional support. The advantages of EN include its stimulatory effects on gastrointestinal structure and function as well as its reduced cost compared to parenteral feeding. Oral nutritional supplements (with 500–600 kcal·day^{-1}) and/or tube feeding improve the nutritional status in adults and especially in children with CD [16]. In fact, 50% of growth-retarded CD patients cannot regain their body weight through medical therapy alone and must use enteral tube feeding [17].

Several studies have demonstrated the efficacy of EN in active CD. While EN's mechanisms of action remain unknown, several hypotheses have been proposed, including the ability of nutrients to modulate the commensal microflora and the intestinal immune response by reducing antigen exposure. In fact, EN seems to exert a direct antiinflammatory effect on the intestinal mucosa by reducing IL-6 production and increasing insulin-like growth factor (IGF)-1 production [18]. However, EN has been proven to be effective in the treatment of the acute phase of CD, achieving remission rates from 20% to 84.2% regardless of disease location. The variability in these results may stem from differences among study populations, administration protocols and outcome assessments [12].

To date, no definitive data has been published on supplementation with oral nutritional supplements in UC patients, who should undergo enteral tube feeding only in exceptional cases [12].

2.2.1. Oral Nutritional Supplementation

Patients with IBD often report concern that their diet may exacerbate their symptoms, and many modify their diet in the hope of controlling symptoms or preventing relapse [19].

This becomes a concern when patients drastically reduce or completely avoid nutritionally important foods, which may put them at risk of developing nutritional deficiencies. Most patients believe that diet influenced their disease and modify their diet. The most common behaviour is the avoidance of milk and dairy products; this dietary change resulted in reduced calcium intakes but had no apparent effect on the rate of relapse [20,21].

Moreover, the exclusion of fruit and vegetables is common (legumes 29.5%; vegetables 18% and fruit 11%) [21]. Unnecessary dietary exclusions, particularly of milk and dairy products, are a concern if initiated without appropriate nutritional or medical supervision.

Although some data suggest that dietary factors play a role in the onset and the course of IBD, recommendations other than following a healthy and varied diet cannot currently be made for most patients [22]. Prescribing a low-residue diet, low in insoluble fiber, may be advisable during acute flares of IBD, particularly in patients with stricturing CD or severe UC attacks [23]. Recently, several hypotheses about the possibility that some specific nutrients can modulate inflammation have been suggested. Specifically, the anti-inflammatory effects of *n*-3 (omega-3 fatty acids, fish oil) have been suggested to be beneficial in chronic inflammatory disorders such as inflammatory bowel disease [24]. At present, data are available mainly on the beneficial effect of *n*-3 polyunsaturated fatty acids (PUFAs) and fermentable fiber [22].

Fermentable fiber generates much less residue than insoluble fiber, and it is fermented by colonic microflora, yielding several products, such as butyrate, than can be beneficial for IBD. Butyrate is the main metabolic substrate for colonic epithelial cells, and there is *in vitro* evidence suggesting that butyrate is able to down-regulate the production of pro-inflammatory cytokines, to promote the restoration of intracellular reactive oxygen species (ROS) balance and the activation of NF-κB [25].

2.2.2. Enteral Tube Feeding

The mechanism underlying a therapeutic response to enteral diets remain unclear [19]. Initially, it was thought that a low antigenic load (absence of whole protein) in the elemental diet was responsible for inducing remission—but it is now known that whole protein enteral feeds are as effective as elemental diets [26]. One of the theories that offers the most exciting possibilities concerns the potential anti-inflammatory effect of an enteral diet on the gastrointestinal mucosa [27]. This may be related to the provision of fatty acids in the feed [28] and/or the potential of the feed to alter gut flora. There is now stronger evidence that the clinical response to an enteral diet is accompanied by histological healing of the mucosa and down regulation of mucosal pro-inflammatory cytokines [27].

Enteral feeding is largely free from side effects. Minor side effects may occur and nausea and headaches may be reported, but these usually resolve after the first few days of feeding. Gradual introduction of the feed during the initial 3–4 days should limit diarrhea. Weight loss, abdominal cramps and vomiting can also occur but they usually resolve as the patient adapts to the diet. The main problems with this regime are often related to poor compliance and unpalatability. These problems may be improved by administering this therapy as part of a multidisciplinary team approach involving the medical, dietetic and nursing staff, as well as the patient and family members, and providing support and education. It is important to acknowledge that exclusive enteral nutrition can, understandably, be a demanding and difficult therapy for many patients [19].

Patients should receive 25–35 kcal·kg^{-1}·day^{-1} by continuous infusion via a nasogastric tube. Infusion rates over 120 mL·h^{-1} frequently lead to diarrhea or reflux. To limit the infusion rate, nutrition should be infused 24 h a day.

It is useful to start enteral nutrition at a low infusion rate of 20 mL h^{-1} and increase this over 2–3 days to the full dose. Additionally, in many patients who are dehydrated due to severe diarrhea, electrolyte solutions have to be infused parenterally during the first few days.

Enteral nutrition should be continued for a minimum of two and preferably four weeks. The dose and duration is dependent on clinical parameters like nutritional status and decrease in disease activity. When symptoms improve, the patient may be allowed some additional food and enteral nutrition may be reduced, dovetailing with the increase in oral nutrition [10].

2.3. Home Enteral Nutrition (HEN)

The most common home infusion therapy today is home enteral nutrition (HEN) or home enteral tube feeding (HETF). HEN should be used in patients who cannot meet their nutrient requirements by oral intake but have a functional gastrointestinal tract, and who are able to receive therapy outside of an acute care setting. It is estimated that more than 300,000 people of all ages in the USA are receiving enteral nutrition at home, whereas in Europe, HETF in the community has also considerably increased in the last few years [29]. Epidemiologic data from UK show that, at any one time, over 19,500 patients receive HETF in the UK community, more than twice that in hospitals [30].

Several factors have contributed to the rapid growth of HEN, including increased awareness of therapeutic nutrition, developments in artificial nutrition, a higher proportion of elderly people in the population, and reduction in the number of hospital beds.

Gastrostomy and/or jejunostomy feeding tubes are frequently inserted and used for long-term home enteral nutrition support. Although insertion of these tubes is usually related to minor morbidity, their long-term use may contribute to various complications and problems which may affect quality of life and have significant economic consequences on health care use [29].

Percutaneous endoscopic gastrostomy (PEG) is actually indicated for patients requiring long-term nutritional support (>30 day) who have a functional gastrointestinal tract but insufficient oral intake of nutrients. There are three techniques for PEG tube placement: the peroral pull technique, the peroral push technique and the direct percutaneous procedure [31]. The most widely-used technique for PEG placement is the "pull" method introduced by Gauderer *et al.* in 1980 [32], which has replaced surgical gastrostomy as the medium- and long-term solution to enteral nutrition delivery, being safer and more cost-effective, with lower procedure-related mortality (0.5%–2%). Furthermore, tube displacement occurs less frequently than with nasogastric tubes [31].

Long-term jejunal feeding can be achieved endoscopically with jejunal tubes through the PEG (JET-PEG) and direct percutaneous endoscopic jejunostomy (DPEJ). Jejunal feeding is appropriate for patients with recurrent vomiting and/or tube feeding-related aspiration, severe gastroesophageal reflux, gastroparesis, gastric outlet obstruction, or total or partial gastrectomy [31].

A complication related to PEG tubes is the formation of gastrocolic, colocutaneous or gastrocolocutaneous fistulae, especially in IBD patients with an active disease. In contrast to the gastrocolic fistula, a fistulous passage connecting the stomach with the colon, the gastrocolocutaneous fistula is defined as an epithelial connection between the mucosa of the stomach, the colon, and the skin. Its probable etiology is the penetration of a bowel loop (mostly transverse colon) interposed between the stomach and the abdominal wall, either by inadvertent puncture during tube placement or, more commonly, due to gradual erosion of the tube into the adjacent bowel [33].

3. Complications of Enteral Tube Feeding

Despite the overall safety of feeding tubes, a number of complications can occur following their placement, though they are usually considered minor, including tube dislodgment, peristomal leakage, and wound infection [34,35]; also, most studies have suggested that complications are more likely to occur in elderly patients with comorbid illnesses, particularly those with an infectious process or who have a history of aspiration [36].

Nevertheless, enteral tube feeding is considered "routine" by many health care professionals involved with it, because these tubes are the most common and easiest to manage in the community. However, as tube feeding can still be a daunting thought for patients and caregivers, careful consideration should be given to predischarge planning and training. Planning for discharge on HEN should begin at the earliest opportunity and involve all the relevant health care professionals and community staff [37], while discussing with the patients and caregivers what to expect on a daily basis when administering HEN [38]. Also, training patients and/or caregivers on caring for the tube, hygiene issues, safety, and basic problem solving is of paramount importance, and they must be clear regarding arrangements for supply of feed and equipment. Consequently, by the time of discharge, patients and caregivers should be adequately trained on the various aspects of the tube feeding system, to ensure safe and effective feeding at home [29].

As tube dysfunction is the most frequent complication related to its presence, some simple measures must be taken to prevent or, at least, to decrease its incidence. For example, tubes may become clogged or occluded if not flushed with water after each feeding, or feedings may leak around the exit site of the tube if tube is too loose, if the balloon is broken, if the tract is enlarged, or the stomach too full. Consequently, the placement of the tube must be frequently checked, and it must be resecured to keep it in place [29].

Recently, it was demonstrated that using a nasal bridle can decrease inadvertent removal of nasally inserted enteral tubes and improve subsequent patient outcomes. The use of the bridles may be benefical in patients with conditions that limit the effectiveness of traditional tubes [39].

4. Conclusions

Enteral nutrition should be used as primary therapy in CD for a number of reasons. First, it fulfils the therapeutic criteria for use in a wide group of patients with CD, since it achieves equal or higher remission rates than some of the drugs currently used. At the same time, it is free of the aesthetic, haematologic, systemic and metabolic side effects commonly associated with steroids and other immune modulators. In addition, in some cases, mucosal healing has been demonstrated with this therapy. Second, enteral nutrition treats or prevents nutritional deficits associated with IBD. It also enhances growth and sexual development in children and adolescents and partly prevents or reverses osteopenia. Enteral nutrition should be the treatment of choice for children and adolescents, not only for the first attack but also for any relapse and as maintenance therapy. Similarly, it should be seen as the first possible treatment for elderly patients with CD in order to maintain their bone mass, since there is a strong possibility that they may have received various long-term treatments with glucocorticoids during their life. Third, enteral formulas should be tried for new onset attacks of CD at all ages to avoid steroid side effects. It should also be the first therapeutic approach in all mild to moderate acute attacks, in particular when there is small intestine or ileocolonic involvement. Finally, a further advantage of this approach is that it is a safer way of starting the treatment in patients with a possible undiagnosed abdominal abscess [2].

Author Contributions: R.A. wrote the manuscript, A.A., G.D. and S.B. contributed to the writing, G.D. and V.D.P. reviewed the manuscript, and A.I.L. and G.T. provided guidance and scientific oversight to the development of the manuscript.

Conflicts of Interest: The authors declare no conflict of interest.

References

1. De Sousa, R.L.M.; Ferreira, S.M.R.; Schieferdecker, M.E.M. Physicochemical and nutricional characteristics of handmade enteral diets. *Nutr. Hosp.* **2014**, *29*, 568–574.
2. Gassull, M.A. New insights in nutritional therapy in inflammatory bowel disease. *Clin. Nutr.* **2001**, *20*, 113–121.
3. Van Heel, D.A.; Satsangi, J.; Carey, A.H.; Jewell, D.P. Inflammatory bowel disease: Progress toward a gene. *Can. J. Gastroenterol.* **2000**, *14*, 207–218.
4. Jones, V.A.; Workman, E.; Wilson, A.J.; Freeman, A.H.; Dickinson, R.J.; Hunter, J.U. Crohn's disease: Maintenance of remission by diet. *Lancet* **1985**, *2*, 177–180.
5. Gassull, M.A.; Abad, A.; Cabrè, E.; Gonzfilez-Huix, F.; Ginè, J.J.; Dolz, C. Enteral tube feeding in inflammatory bowel disease. *Gut* **1986**, *27*, 76–80.
6. O'Morain, C.; Segal, A.W.; Levi, A.J. Elemental diet as primary treatment of acute Crohn's disease: A controlled study. *BMJ* **1984**, *228*, 1859–1862.
7. Teahon, K.; Smethurst, P.; Pearson, M.; Levi, A.J.; Bjarnason, I. The effect of elemental diet on intestinal permeability and inflammation in Crohn's disease. *Gastroenterology* **1991**, *101*, 84–89.
8. Lochs, H.; Dejong, C.; Hammarqvist, F.; Hebuterne, X.; Leon-Sanz, M.; Schütz, T. ESPEN Guidelines on Enteral Nutrition: Gastroenterology. *Clin. Nutr.* **2006**, *25*, 260–274.
9. Van Gossum, A.; Cabre, E.; Hébuterne, X.; Jeppesen, P.; Krznaric, Z.; Messing, B. ESPEN Guidelines on Parental Nutrition: Gastroenterology. *Clin. Nutr.* **2009**, *28*, 415–427.
10. Lochs, H. Basics in Clinical Nutrition: Nutritional support in inflammatory bowel disease. *Eur. e-J. Clin. Nutr. Met.* **2010**, *5*, 100–103. Available online: http://www.sciencedirect.com/science/journal/17514991/5/2 (accessed on 9 June 2009).
11. Yao, G.X.; Wang, X.R.; Jiang, Z.M.; Zhang, S.Y.; Ni, A.P. Role of perioperative parenteral nutrition in severely malnourished patients with Crohn's disease. *World J. Gastroenterol.* **2005**, *11*, 5732–5734.
12. Guagnozzi, D.; González-Castillo, S.; Olveira, A.; Lucendo, A.J. Nutritional treatment in inflammatory bowel disease. An update. *Rev. Esp. Enferm. Dig.* **2012**, *104*, 479–488.
13. Wild, G.E.; Drozdowski, L.; Tartaglia, C.; Clandinin, M.T.; Thomson, A.B.R. Nutritional modulation of the inflammatory response in inflammatory bowel disease-from the molecular to the integrative to the clinical. *World J. Gastroenterol.* **2007**, *13*, 1–7.
14. Scolapio, J.S. The role of total parenteral nutrition in the management of patients with acute attacks of inflammatory bowel disease. *J. Clin. Gastroenterol.* **1999**, *29*, 223–224.
15. Ostro, M.J.; Greenberg, G.; Jeejeebhoy, K.N. Total parenteral nutrition and complete bowel rest in the management of Crohn's disease. *J. Parenter. Enteral. Nutr.* **1985**, *9*, 280–287.
16. Harries, A.D.; Jones, L.A.; Danis, V.; Fifield, R.; Heatley, R.V.; Newcombe, R.G. Controlled trial of supplemented oral nutrition in Crohn's disease. *Lancet* **1983**, *1*, 887–890.

17. Motil, K.J.; Grand, R.J.; Davis-Kraft, L.; Ferlic, L.L.; Smith, E.O. Growth failure in children with inflammatory bowel disease: A prospective study. *Gastroenterology* **1993**, *105*, 681–691.

18. Bannerjee, K.; Camacho-Hübner, C.; Babinsk, K.; Dryhurst, K.M.; Edwards, R.; Savage, M.O. Anti-inflammatory and growth-stimulating effects precede nutritional restitution during enteral feeding in Crohn's disease. *J. Pedriatr. Gastroenterol. Nutr.* **2004**, *38*, 270–275.

19. O'Sullivan, M. Nutrition in inflammatory bowel disease. *Best Pract. Res. Clin. Gastroenterol.* **2006**, *20*, 561–573.

20. Jowett, S.L.; Seal, C.J.; Phillips, E. Dietary beliefs of people with ulcerative colitis and their effect on relapse and nutrient intake. *Clin. Nutr.* **2004**, *23*, 161–170.

21. Guerreiro, C.; Valonqueiro, A.; Costa, M. Dietary changes in patients with Crohn's Disease (CD): Impact in macro and micronutient intake. *Clin. Nutr.* **2005**, *24*, 636.

22. Massironi, S.; Rossi, R.E.; Cavalcoli, F.A.; Della Valle, S.; Fraquelli, M.; Conte, D. Nutritional deficiencies in inflammatory bowel disease: Therapeutic approaches. *Clin. Nutr.* **2013**, *32*, 904–910.

23. Cabré, E.; Domènech, E. Impact of environmental and dietary factors on the course of inflammatory bowel disease. *World J. Gastroenterol.* **2012**, *18*, 3814–3822.

24. Turner, D.; Zlotkin, S.H.; Shah, P.S.; Griffiths, A.M. Omega 3 fatty acids (fish oil) for maintenance of remission in Crohn's disease. *The Cochrane Libr.* **2009**, *1*. [CrossRef]

25. Russo, I.; Luciani, A.; De Cicco, P.; Troncone, E.; Ciacci, C. Butyrate attenuates lipopolysaccharide-induced inflammation in intestinal cells and Crohn's mucosa through modulation of antioxidant defense machinery. *PLoS ONE* **2012**, *7*, e32841.

26. Verma, S.; Brown, S.; Kirkwood, B.; Giaffer, M. Polymeric versus elemental diet as primary treatment in active Crohn's disease: A randomized, double-blind trial. *Am. J. Gastroenterol.* **2000**, *95*, 735–739.

27. Fell, J.M.; Paintin, M.; Arnaud-Battandier, F. Mucosal healing and a fall in mucosal pro-inflammatory cytokine mRNA induced by a specific oral polymeric diet in paediatric Crohn's disease. *Aliment. Pharm. Ther.* **2000**, *14*, 281–289.

28. Gassull, M.A.; Fernandez-Banares, F.; Cabre, E. Fat composition may be a clue to explain the primary therapeutic effect of enteral nutrition in Crohn's disease: Results of a double blind randomised multicentre European trial. *Gut* **2002**, *51*, 164–168.

29. Alivizatos, V.; Gavala, V.; Alexopoulos, P.; Apostolopoulos, A.; Bajrucevic, S. Feeding Tube-related Complications and Problems in Patients Receiving Longterm Home Enteral Nutrition. *Indian J. Pall. Care* **2012**, *18*, 31–33.

30. Madigan, S.M.; Fleming, P.; McCann, S.; Wright, M.E.; MacAuley, D. General Practitioners involvement in enteral tube feeding at home: A qualitative study. *BMC Fam. Pract.* **2007**, *8*, 29.

31. Blumestein, I.; Shastri, Y.M.; Stein, J. Gastroenteric tube feeding: Techniques, problems and solutions. *World J. Gastroent.* **2014**, *20*, 8505–8524.

32. Gauderer, M.W.; Ponsky, J.L.; Izant, R.J. Gastrostomy without laparotomy: A percutaneous endoscopic technique. *J. Pediatr. Surg.* **1980**, *15*, 872–875.

33. Berger, S.A.; Zarling, E.J. Colocutaneous fistula following migration of PEG tube. *Gastrointest. Endocr.* **1991**, *37*, 86–88.

34. Taylor, C.A.; Larson, D.E.; Ballard, D.J.; Bergstrom, L.R.; Silverstein, M.D.; Zinsmeister, A.R. Predictors of outcome after percutaneous endoscopic gastrostomy: A community-based study. *Mayo Clin. Proc.* **1992**, *67*, 1042–1049.

35. Larson, D.E.; Burton, D.D.; Schroeder, K.W.; Di Magno, E.P. Percutaneous endoscopic gastrostomy. Indications, success, complications and mortality in 314 consecutive patients. *Gastroentrology* **1987**, *93*, 48–52.

36. Raha, S.K.; Woodhouse, K. The use of percutaneous endoscopic gastrostomy (PEG) in 161 consecutive elderly patients. *Age Ageing* **1994**, *23*, 162–163.

37. Mensforth, A.; Spelding, D. Discharge planning for home enteral tube feeding. *Clin. Nutr. Update* **1998**, *3*, 8–10.

38. Goff, K. Enteral and parenteral nutrition transitioning from hospital to home. *Nurs. Case. Manag.* **1998**, *3*, 67–74.

39. Parks, J.; Klaus, S.; Staggs, V.; Pena, M. Outcomes of nasal bridling to secure enteral tubes in burn patients. *Am. J. Crit. Care* **2013**, *22*, 136–142.

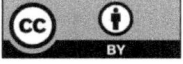

nutrients

Review

Enteral Nutrition in Dementia: A Systematic Review

Joanne Brooke [1,*] and Omorogieva Ojo [2]

[1]   Kent Community Health NHS Trust, The Oast, Unit D, Maidstone Kent ME16 9NT, UK
[2]   School of Health and Social Care, Faculty of Education and Health, University of Greenwich, Avery Hill Campus, London SE9 2UG, UK; o.ojo@greenwich.ac.uk
*   Author to whom correspondence should be addressed; joanne.brooke@kentcht.nhs.uk; Tel.: +44-(0)1622-211-920.

Received: 25 November 2014; Accepted: 27 March 2015; Published: 3 April 2015

Abstract: The aim of this systematic review is to evaluate the role of enteral nutrition in dementia. The prevalence of dementia is predicted to rise worldwide partly due to an aging population. People with dementia may experience both cognitive and physical complications that impact on their nutritional intake. Malnutrition and weight loss in dementia correlates with cognitive decline and the progress of the disease. An intervention for long term eating difficulties is the provision of enteral nutrition through a Percutaneous Endoscopic Gastrostomy tube to improve both nutritional parameters and quality of life. Enteral nutrition in dementia has traditionally been discouraged, although further understanding of physical, nutritional and quality of life outcomes are required. The following electronic databases were searched: EBSCO Host, MEDLINE, PubMed, Cochrane Database of Systematic Reviews and Google Scholar for publications from 1st January 2008 and up to and including 1st January 2014. Inclusion criteria included the following outcomes: mortality, aspiration pneumonia, pressure sores, nutritional parameters and quality of life. Each study included separate analysis for patients with a diagnosis of dementia and/or neurological disease. Retrospective and prospective observational studies were included. No differences in mortality were found for patients with dementia, without dementia or other neurological disorders. Risk factors for poor survival included decreased or decreasing serum albumin levels, increasing age or over 80 years and male gender. Evidence regarding pneumonia was limited, although did not impact on mortality. No studies explored pressure sores or quality of life.

Keywords: enteral nutrition; dementia; percutaneous endoscopic gastrostomy; nasogastric tube; serum albumin

1. Introduction

Due to a global aging population the incidence and prevalence of dementia is predicted to rise worldwide, with an estimated 81 million people diagnosed with dementia by 2040 [1]. Dementia is an umbrella term for a number of specific conditions which are progressive in nature and impact on multiple areas of functioning including decline in memory, reasoning, communication skills and ability to carry out daily activities [2].

A common experience for people with dementia is the development of eating difficulties leading to problems such as malnutrition and weigh loss [3,4]. The severity and progression of dementia is closely related to weight loss [5,6]. In the early stages of dementia eating difficulties are attributed to olfactory and taste dysfunction, executive planning difficulties, attention deficits, dyspraxia, agnosia and behavioural problems [7]. In advanced stages of dementia oral and pharyngeal phase dysphagia may be present leading to the inability to coordinate chewing and swallowing, and disruption of the food bolus from the oropharynx into the oesophagus without aspiration [8]. Reduced nutrition has negative outcomes for patients with dementia including higher morbidity and mortality, reduced quality of life and increased carer burden [9–11].

An intervention for long term eating difficulties across different health conditions is the provision of enteral nutrition through a Percutaneous Endoscopic Gastrostomy (PEG) tube. The provision of enteral nutrition is both to provide complete nutrition and improve the patient's quality of life [12]. A systematic review in 1999 explored the impact of enteral nutrition in patients with advanced dementia and found no improvements in the rates of aspiration, pressures sores or mortality [13]. No data was found on quality of life, although many complications were reported including: gastric perforation, gastric prolapse, aspiration, diarrhoea, gastrointestinal bleeding, nauseas and vomiting, fluid overload and loss of social aspects of feeding. Finucane *et al.* [13] concluded enteral nutrition for patients with dementia should be actively discouraged.

A further review in 2001 explored nutritional parameters, quality of life and mortality of older people with dementia receiving enteral nutrition [14]. A small number of studies (*n* = 3) found improvements in nutritional parameters and an increased albumin was associated with decreased mortality. Dharmarajan *et al.* [14] found quality of life was difficult to analyse in this population as patients with advanced dementia could not narrate their subjective feelings, and family members reported conflicting opinions. Mortality ranged from 11%–27% across studies at 30 days post insertion of a PEG and commencement of enteral nutrition. However, mortality was not uniformed: older patients, men and patients with an acute illness had higher mortality than women and African-American patients. Dharmarajan *et al.* [14] recommended caution in decisions regarding enteral nutrition in older people with dementia.

A more recent review in 2009 reported no significant association between enteral nutrition and decreased mortality in older patients with dementia [15]. Secondary outcomes of weight loss, Body Mass Index (BMI), haemocrit and cholesterol were not significantly different between those receiving enteral nutrition to those who were not, albumin levels were significantly decreased in patients receiving enteral nutrition [15]. No studies in this review explored the impact of enteral nutrition on quality of life, behavioural or psychiatric symptoms of dementia. However, one study documented the use of restraint, with 71% of patients being physically restrained to prevent removal of a PEG compared to 55% of those not receiving enteral nutrition [16]. Sampson *et al.* [15] conclude that there is insufficient evidence to suggest enteral nutrition in patients with advanced dementia is beneficial.

Clinical guidance reflects the evidence to date, National Institute for Health and Care Excellence (NICE) guidance [17] suggests enteral nutrition may be considered if dysphagia in a patient with dementia is deemed to be transient, but should not generally be used for patients with advanced dementia who are disinclined to eat or have permanent dysphagia. European Society of Parenteral and Enteral Nutrition (ESPEN) are shortly to realise their guidelines on Nutrition in Dementia [7]. ESPEN confirm the use of enteral nutrition in patients with mild or moderate dementia if malnutrition is predominantly the cause of a reversible condition and only for a limited time. Reversible conditions are secondary concurrent illnesses such as depression, infection, over use of sedatives, pain or poor oral health. ESPEN do not recommend the use of enteral nutrition in the terminal phase of dementia, although acknowledge decisions are unique for each patient with dementia and should take into consideration the patient's general prognosis and preferences.

Decisions regarding enteral nutrition in advanced dementia remain ethically challenging for all involved [4]. One challenge is the possible complications of enteral nutrition including aspiration pneumonia and fluid overload [13,18]. Further challenges include understanding the patient's wishes as they may be unable to communicate and are unlikely to have documented their wishes through advance directives or advance care plans [19,20].

However, evidence suggests the continued use of enteral nutrition in the older population with dementia. A study in the United States found 34% of nursing home residents received enteral nutrition [21] and 30% of PEG insertions were estimated to be in people with dementia [22]. In Japan, elderly people receiving enteral nutrition is on the increase [23]. Many studies and reviews have been completed exploring the immediate clinical effects of enteral nutrition for people with advanced dementia [13–15,24]. However, methodologies, focus and outcomes of these studies have begun to change and the need to explore further risk factors for patients with dementia receiving enteral nutrition is required. Therefore the aim of this review is to explore recent data on both physical and nutritional outcomes and the impact on quality of life of patients with dementia receiving enteral nutrition.

Objectives:

- Evaluate the impact of enteral nutrition on mortality, risk factors for mortality, pressure sores, aspiration pneumonia and nutritional parameters for patients with dementia.
- Evaluate the impact of enteral nutrition on quality of life for patients with dementia.

2. Experimental Section

Published guidelines [25,26] were used to complete a systematic review. An initial scoping exercise identified three relevant systematic reviews [13–15], which informed the criteria for the search. The following electronic databases were searched: EBSCO Host, MEDLINE, PubMed, Cochrane Database of Systematic Reviews and Google Scholar for publications from 1st January 2008 and up to and including 1st January 2014. Search words included *enteral nutrition, enteral feeding, artificial nutrition, artificial nutrition, percutaneous endoscopic gastrostomy* and *dementia*, with *and/or* Boolean operators (refer to Table 1 Literature Search Strategy). All searchers were limited to "English Language". In addition bibliographies of identified articles were manually searched for relevant studies.

Nutrients **2015**, *7*, 2456–2468

Table 1. Literature Search Strategy.

Key Words	Search Engine	Hits	Search Engine	Hits	Search Engine	Hits	Search Engine	Hits	Search Engine	Hits
enteral nutrition 'and' dementia	EBSCO Host	168	PubMed	100	MEDLINE	317	COCHRANE DATABASE	3	GOOGLE SCHOLAR	5630
enteral feeding 'and' dementia	EBSCO Host	62	PubMed	102	MEDLINE	324	COCHRANE DATABASE	3	GOOGLE SCHOLAR	4380
enteral feeding 'and' dementia patients	EBSCO Host	13	PubMed	63	MEDLINE	324	COCHRANE DATABASE	3	GOOGLE SCHOLAR	4510
artificial nutrition 'and' dementia	EBSCO Host	96	PubMed	39	MEDLINE	98	COCHRANE DATABASE	1	GOOGLE SCHOLAR	14,300
nasogastric tube 'and' dementia	EBSCO Host	14	PubMed	0	MEDLINE	38	COCHRANE DATABASE	2	GOOGLE SCHOLAR	16,100
percutaneous endoscopic gastrostomy 'and' dementia	EBSCO Host	2	PubMed	78	MEDLINE	124	COCHRANE DATABASE	2	GOOGLE SCHOLAR	2330
artificial feeding 'and' dementia	EBSCO Host	30	PubMed	354	MEDLINE	947	COCHRANE DATABASE	1	GOOGLE SCHOLAR	18,500

2.1. Inclusion and Exclusion Criteria

In addition to the search strategy above the inclusion criteria were: measured outcomes of mortality, aspiration pneumonia, pressure sores, nutritional parameters and quality of life, and a separate analysis of patients with a primary diagnosis of dementia or neurological disease. Exclusion criteria were: administration of enteral nutrition via nasogastric tubes, intravenous fluids and short term interventions. Two studies were excluded as analysis combined the outcomes of patients with dementia receiving enteral nutrition via a nasogastric tubes and PEG tubes [27,28].

3. Results

A total of five studies were included in the systematic review and all had an observational design. Two studies applied a prospective design [29,30] and three studies applied a retrospective design [31–33]. Studies were completed in Japan [31], USA [32], Sweden [29,33] and Germany [30]. Study sample sizes ranged from 119–484, participants were categorized with a diagnosis of dementia [31,33] or a broader definition of dementia as significant cognitive impairment and/or combined with other neurologic disorders [29,30,32]. All studies included enteral nutrition administered via PEG tubes. All studies included mortality following the commencement of enteral nutrition or the insertion of a PEG. Mortality was analysed using Kapan-Meirer analysis, which is an estimate of the number of participants who survive for a certain amount of time following a healthcare intervention [34]. Secondary outcomes included predictors of mortality, serum albumin levels, aspiration pneumonia and general complications. No studies reported outcomes relevant to pressure sores or quality of life (refer to Table 2 Summary of studies reviewed).

3.1. Mortality

Kaplan-Meirer survival analysis were completed by all five studies [29–33]. No significant differences in mortality were demonstrated in two studies when patients with dementia were compared to those without dementia or other neurological conditions [31–33]. Decreased mortality for patients with dementia was demonstrated by one study when compared to patients with stroke, malignant diseases and other neurological conditions [33]. Increased mortality for patients with dementia and other neurological diseases was a significant finding in two studies [20,30] when compared to patients with tumours.

3.2. Predictors of Mortality

A low or decreasing serum albumin was a predictive factor of increased mortality in three studies [29,31,32]. Increasing age, or age over 80 years were predictive factors of increased mortality in four studies [29,31–33]. Further risk factors identified by individual studies included male [31], an additional diagnosis of chronic heart failure [31] and a raised CRP [29].

3.3. Pressure Sores

No studies included in the review explored the impact of enteral nutrition and pressure sore development and healing.

3.4. Aspiration Pneumonia

Pneumonia including aspiration pneumonia was explored by three studies [30–32]. Rates of pneumonia whilst receiving enteral nutrition via a PEG tube was 5% and was not a risk factor of mortality [30–32]. One study reported aspiration pneumonia rates were comparable across patients with dementia and those without dementia receiving enteral nutrition [31]. One study reported pneumonia rates, not linked to aspiration were comparable across patients with neurologic conditions and tumours receiving enteral nutrition.

3.5. Quality of Life

No studies included in the review explored the impact of enteral nutrition and quality of life for patients with dementia.

Table 2. Summary of Studies Reviewed.

Author	Study, Design, Country of Study	Population Size	Age Mean SD	Kaplan-Meier Survival Analysis	Predictors for Poor Survival
Higaki *et al.* 2008 [31]	Retrospective study of PEG enteral nutrition Compared outcomes of patients with and without dementia in the elderly Japan	311 46.0% (n = 143) with dementia 54.0% (n = 168) without dementia 78.8	83.7 ± 8 with dementia 78.8 ± 11 without dementia	No significant difference in mortality between patients with dementia and those without dementia (p = 0.62)	-subtotal gastrectomy (OR 2.619, 95% CI: 1.367–5.019) -serum albumin <2.8 g/dL (OR 2.081, 95% CI: 1.490–2.905) -age > 80 years (OR 1.721, 95% CI: 1.234–2.399) -chronic heart failure (OR 1.541, 95% CI: 1.096–2.168) -male (OR 1.407, 95% CI: 1.037–1.909)
Gaines *et al.* 2009 [32]	Retrospective study of PEG enteral nutrition Compared outcomes for patients with dementia or significant cognitive impairment (SCI) to those without these conditions USA	190 23.7% (n = 45) dementia or SCI 76.3% (n = 145) without dementia or SCI	Median age: 64	No significant difference in mortality in patients with dementia or SCI and those without (p = 0.85)	Predictors for 30-day mortality -increasing age (OR 1.08, 95% CI: 1.04–1.12) -decreasing serum albumin (OR 0.43, 95% CI: 0.22–0.84)
Malmgren *et al.* 2011 [33]	Retrospective study of PEG enteral nutrition Indications for survival after PEG insertion in patients older than 65 Sweden	191 8.4% (n = 16) dementia 5.8% (n = 11) Parkinson 9.5% (n = 19) miscellaneous 49.7% (n = 95) stroke 18.4% (n = 35) malignant 6.8% (n = 13) neurological diseases	79.0 ± 7	Patients with dementia or Parkinsons had longest median survival	-patients with dementia >80 years of age than those with dementia <80 years of age (p = 0.025)
Blomberg *et al.* 2012 [29]	Observational prospective study of PEG enteral nutrition Outcome of patients following PEG insertion Sweden	484 44% (n = 214) tumours 45% (n = 218) neurological disease including dementia	66.0 ± 14	Mortality higher in patients with neurological disorders than those with tumours (p = 0.002)	-serum albumin < 30 g/L (hazard ration (HR), 3.46; 95% CI 1.75–6.88) -CRP ≥ 10 (HR, 3.47; 95% CI 1.68–7.18) -age ≥ 65 (HR, 2.26; 95% CI 1.20–4.25)
Schneider *et al.* 2014 [30]	Observational prospective study of PEG enteral nutrition Outcomes of patients following PEG insertion Germany	119 57.2% (n = 68) tumours 29.4% (n = 35) neurologic including dementia 13.4% (16) other	63.0 ± 13	Mortality higher in patients with neurological disorders than those with tumours (p = 0.002)	NA

4. Discussion

In this review, the impact of enteral nutrition on mortality was equivalent for patients with dementia, without dementia or diagnosed with other neurological conditions. However, patients with dementia had decreased mortality compared to patients with a stroke and increased mortality compared to patients with tumours. Risk factors for poor survival included decreased or decreasing serum albumin levels, increasing age or over 80 years, and male gender. Limited evidence on pneumonia was found, although did not impacted on mortality. No studies explored the development or healing of pressure sores or quality of life.

Previous studies have failed to demonstrate enteral nutrition for patients with dementia prolongs survival [18,35–37]. Current studies suggest mortality of patients with dementia receiving enteral nutrition when compared to other conditions is dependent on the comparativeness of these conditions, including stage of the disease and long term prognosis. The importance of the timing of the decision with regards to the prognosis of the patient with dementia may be an influential factor, as enteral nutrition is more frequently commenced in advanced dementia [33]. Patients with advanced dementia may exhibit a low level of functionality over a long period of time, which contributes to general frailty [38]. Illness trajectories and mortality in dementia are difficult to predict due to low functionality and frailty, which leads to discussions regarding enteral nutrition in the advanced stages of dementia as end of life is difficult to recognize [38,39]. Therefore, the possibility of some studies to include older patients with more advanced dementia and the tendency to commence enteral nutrition in the late stages of the disease process may have implications for mortality rates.

In the current review a decreased or decreasing serum albumin was a predictor of mortality [29, 31,32]. Decreased serum albumin levels (<3.0 mg/dL) have been associated with increased mortality in enteral nutrition where analysis did not differentiate the diagnosis of patients [40,41]. Evidence for the impact of the diagnosis of dementia and decreasing serum albumin levels for patients receiving enteral nutrition is inconsistent. One study found serum albumin levels did not predict survival in patients with dementia, but did predict survival in patients without dementia receiving enteral nutrition [42]. The impact of serum albumin levels in patients not receiving enteral nutrition needs to be considered, as decreased serum albumin in critical illness was associated with increased mortality [43]. In the healthy elderly serum albumin levels decreased with age and were predictive of mortality independent of know disease [44]. Evidence regarding decreased or decreasing serum albumin levels suggests an impact on mortality and therefore, needs to be considered in the provision of enteral nutrition regardless of diagnosis but with consideration of age.

Aspiration pneumonia has been a recognised complication of advanced dementia and enteral nutrition administered via PEG tubes [3]. Finucane *et al.* [13] reported no randomised controlled trials had explored the reduction of aspiration pneumonia following the provision of enteral nutrition via a PEG tube. In the current review one observational study reported aspiration pneumonia occurrence at 5%, which was comparable for patients with and without dementia and was not a risk factor of mortality [31]. Tentatively enteral nutrition delivered through a PEG tube does not increase the risk of aspiration for patients with dementia compared to rates of aspiration pneumonia of other disease cohorts.

The development and healing of pressure sores was not explored by the studies included in this review. However, Martin *et al.* [27] explored the impact of enteral nutrition administered via nasogastric tubes and PEG tubes reported pressure and reported that a fifth of patients developed a pressure sore during the provision of enteral nutrition, and the healing of pressure sores was correlated with increased mortality. The development and lack of healing of pressure sores may correlate with hypoalbuminemia, as this is a risk factor for the development of pressure sores and increases resistance to treatment [45,46]. No further studies have explored the correlation between serum albumin and pressure sores in patients with dementia receiving enteral nutrition. Martin *et al.* [27] reported enteral nutrition in patients with dementia was effective in preserving but not significantly improving serum albumin levels.

Limitations of the studies included in this review need to be acknowledged. Different clinical practices and guidelines across continents may impact on the results of studies included. Practices across continents were difficult to identify only three studies reported PEG placement procedures and none clarified/defined enteral nutrition. Prevalence of enteral nutrition in patients with dementia in Japan may be higher than Western populations due to current guidelines. In Japan guidelines compiled under the supervision of the Japan Gastroenterology Endoscopy Society recommend PEG insertion for patients who cannot maintain their nutrition due to cerebrovascular disease or dementia [47]. The impact of these guidelines may be the earlier insertion of PEG tubes and the commencement of enteral nutrition in patients with dementia leading to longer survival rates [31]. Higaki *et al.* [31] reported survival at 12 months of 51% for patients with dementia of which 20% were still alive three years, compared to 41% of patients with dementia at 12 months in a study completed in Sweden [33]. However, no longitudinal data was reported outside Japan and the challenges to this guidance and Japanese health-care system reforms may impact on this prevalence [28].

Further limitations of the studies include small sample sizes and different categorization of conditions. Dementia was categorized as a separate neurological condition in some studies, but included with other neurological conditions in further studies. Diagnosis was generalised in some studies to those with and without dementia, and more detailed in further studies with all conditions categorized and therefore, direct comparison and interpretation of results is difficult.

Ethical considerations of insertion of a PEG in a patient with dementia are important. ESPEN and NICE guidelines do not recommend enteral nutrition in patients with advanced dementia and only occasionally in patients in the earlier stages of dementia. Enteral nutrition is recommended only to ensure adequate provision of nutritional needs, when under-nutrition is caused by reversible conditions other than the dementia [48]. However, diagnostic overshadowing, a tendency to attribute all symptoms to dementia thereby leaving a co-existing conditions undiagnosed has been recognised and needs to be continually challenged [49].

Alzheimer's Society supports the importance of quality of life rather than length of life. For the person with dementia decreased quality of life has been associated with behavioural and psychological disturbances, but no associations with dysphagia or cognition has been demonstrated to date [50]. A recent a recent review by the Royal College of Physicians suggests the need for reluctance to commence enteral nutrition in dementia, however state this cannot be translated into a blanket ban [51]. A decision-making algorithm integrating medical and ethic dimensions regarding enteral nutrition in dementia has been developed and may be helpful to healthcare professionals faced with this ethical dilemma [52].

5. Conclusions

The studies included in this systematic review challenge the traditional view that enteral nutrition administered through a PEG tube increases mortality in patients with dementia. The recommendations from this review include the need for a holistic assessment of patients with dementia when contemplating PEG insertion and enteral nutrition. A holistic assessment would include: the patients' diagnosis including comorbidities, current stage and impact of dementia on the need for enteral nutrition, age and nutritional parameters. The impact of enteral nutrition on quality of life for patients with dementia remains unclear, although complications are acknowledged. Enteral nutrition within end of life care is not recommended, although this review acknowledges recognising end of life within dementia is problematic. A further recommendation is early discussions with patients with dementia and their family regarding nutrition needs in advanced dementia and the documentation of the results of these discussions. However, decision making regarding PEG insertion and enteral nutrition in patients with dementia currently remains ethically challenging and should involve discussions around appropriate end of life care.

Author Contributions: Both authors contributed significantly in all aspects of the manuscript, they both read and approved the final copy.

Nutrients **2015**, *7*, 2456–2468

Conflicts of Interest: The authors declare no conflict of interest.

References

1. Ferri, C.P.; Prince, M.; Brayne, C.; Brodaty, H.; Fratiglioni, L.; Ganguli, M.; Hall, K.; Hasegawa, K.; Hendrie, H.; Huang, Y.; *et al.* Global prevalence of dementia: A Delphi consensus study. *Lancet* **2005**, *366*, 2112–2117. [CrossRef] [PubMed]
2. Department of Health. Living well with dementia: A National Dementia Strategy. 2009. Available online: http://tinyurl.com/clcclnz (accessed on 1 July 2014).
3. Mitchell, S.L.; Teno, J.M.; Kiely, D.K.; Shaffer, M.L.; Jones, R.N.; Prigerson, H.G.; Volicer, L.; Givens, J.L.; Hamel, M.B. The clinical course of advanced dementia. *N. Engl. J. Med.* **2009**, *361*, 1529–1538. [CrossRef] [PubMed]
4. Braun, U.K.; Rabeneck, L.; McCullough, L.B.; Urbauer, D.L.; Wray, N.P.; Lairson, D.R.; Beyth, R.J. Decreasing use of Percutaneous Endoscopic Gastrostomy tube feeding for Veterans with dementia-racial differences remain. *J. Am. Geriatr. Soc.* **2005**, *53*, 242–248. [CrossRef] [PubMed]
5. Guerin, S.; Andrieu, S.; Schneider, S.M.; Milano, M.; Boulahssass, R.; Brocker, P.; Vellas, B. Different modes of weight loss in Alzheimer's Disease: A prospective study of 395 patients. *Am. J. Clin. Nutr* **2005**, *82*, 435–441. [PubMed]
6. Spaccavento, S.; de Prete, M.; Craia, A.; Fiore, P. Influence of nutritional status on cognitive, function and neuropsychiatric deficits in Alzheimer's Disease. *Arch. Gerontol. Geriat.* **2009**, *48*, 356–360. [CrossRef]
7. Volkert, D. Guidelines on Nutrition in Dementia. In Proceedings of the 36th ESPEN Congress, Geneva, Switzerland, 9 September 2014.
8. Dodds, W.J.; Stewart, E.T.; Logemann, J.A. Physiology and radiology of the normal oral and pharyngeal phases of swallowing. *AJR* **1990**, *154*, 953–963. [CrossRef] [PubMed]
9. Norman, K.; Pichard, C.; Lochs, H.; Pirlich, M. Prognostic impact of disease-related malnutrition. *Clin. Nutr.* **2008**, *27*, 5–15. [CrossRef] [PubMed]
10. Faxen-Irving, G.; Basum, H.; Cederholm, T. Nutritional and cognitive relationships and long-term mortality in patients with various dementia disorders. *Age Ageing* **2005**, *34*, 136–141. [CrossRef] [PubMed]
11. Ball, L.; Jansen, S.; Desbrow, B.; Morgan, K.; Moyle, W.; Hughes, R. Experiences and nutrition support strategies in dementia care: Lessons from family carers. *Nutr. Diet.* **2014**. [CrossRef]
12. Llyod, D.A.; Powell-Tuck, J. Artificial nutrition: Principals and practice of enteral feeding. *Clin. Colon Rectal Surg.* **2004**, *17*, 107–118. [CrossRef] [PubMed]
13. Finucane, T.E.; Christmas, C.; Travis, K. Tube feeding in patients with advanced dementia: A review of the evidence. *JAMA* **1999**, *282*, 1365–1370. [CrossRef] [PubMed]
14. Dharmarajan, T.S.; Unnikrishnan, D.; Pitchumoni, C.S. Percutaneous endoscopic gastrostomy and outcome in dementia. *Am. J. Gastroenterol.* **2001**, *96*, 2556–2563. [CrossRef] [PubMed]
15. Sampson, E.L.; Candy, B.; Jones, L. Enteral tube feeding for older people with advanced dementia. *Cochrane Database Syst. Rev.* **2009**, *15*, 396–404.
16. Peck, A.; Cohen, C.A.; Mulvihill, M.N. Long-term enteral feeding of aged demented nursing home patients. *J. Am. Geriatr. Soc.* **1990**, *38*, 1195–1198. [PubMed]
17. National Institute for Health and Care Excellence. Dementia: Support People with Dementia and Their Carers in Health and Social Care. 2006. Available online: http://www.nice.org.uk/guidance/cg42/resources/guidance-dementia-pdf (accessed on 1 July 2014).
18. Murphy, L.M.; Lipman, T.O. Percutaneous endoscopic gastrostomy does not prolong survival in patients with dementia. *Arch. Intern. Med.* **2003**, *163*, 1351–1353. [CrossRef] [PubMed]
19. De Boer, M.E.; Hertogh, C.M.; Droes, R.M.; Jonker, C.; Eefsting, J.A. Advance directives in dementia: Issues of validity and effectiveness. *Int. Psychogeriatr.* **2010**, *22*, 201–208. [CrossRef] [PubMed]
20. Brooke, J.; Kirk, M. Advance care planning for people living with dementia. *Br. J. Community Nurs.* **2014**, *19*, 422–427. [CrossRef] [PubMed]
21. Mitchell, S.L.; Teno, J.M.; Roy, L.; Kabumoto, G.; Mor, V. Clinical and organizational factors associated with feeding tube use among nursing home residents with advanced cognitive impairment. *JAMA* **2003**, *290*, 73–80. [CrossRef] [PubMed]

22. Rabeneck, L.; Wray, N.P.; Petersen, N.L. Long-term outcomes of patients receiving percutaneous endoscopic gastrostomy tubes. *J. Gen. Intern. Med.* **1996**, *11*, 287–293. [CrossRef] [PubMed]

23. Kosaka, Y.; Sato, T.; Arai, H. Tube feeding in the bedridden elderly patients. *Nippon Ronen Igakkai Zasshi* **2009**, *46*, 521–523. (In Japanese) [CrossRef] [PubMed]

24. Buiting, H.M.; Clayton, J.M.; Butow, P.N.; van Delden, J.J.M.; van der Heide, A. Artifical nutrition and hydration for patients with advanced dementia: Perspectives from medical practitioners in Netherlands and Australia. *Palliat. Med.* **2011**, *25*, 83–91. [CrossRef] [PubMed]

25. Bettany-Saltikov, J. *How to do a Systematic Literature Review in Nursing*; Ashford Colour Press Ltd.: Gosport, UK, 2012.

26. Wright, R.W.; Brand, R.A.; Dunn, W.; Spindler, K.P. How to write a systematic review. *Clin. Orthop. Relat. Res.* **2007**, *455*, 23–29. [CrossRef] [PubMed]

27. Higaki, F.; Yokota, O.; Ohishi, M. Factors predictive of survival after percutaneous endoscopic gastrostomy in the elderly: Is dementia really a risk factor? *Am. J. Gastroenterol.* **2008**, *103*, 1011–1016. [CrossRef] [PubMed]

28. Gaines, D.I.; Durkalski, V.; Patel, A.; DeLegge, M.H. Dementia and cognitive impairment are not associated with earlier mortality after percutaneous endoscopic gastrostomy. *J. Parenter. Enter. Nutr.* **2009**, *33*, 62–66. [CrossRef]

29. Malmgren, A.; Hede, G.W.; Karlstrom, B.; Cederholm, T.; Lundquist, P.; Wiren, M.; Faxen-Irving, G. Indications for percutaneous endoscopic gastrostomy and survival in old adults. *Food Nutr. Res.* **2011**, *55*, 6037. [CrossRef]

30. Martins, A.L.; de Rezende, N.A.; da Gama Torres, H.Q. Occurrence of complications and survival rates in elderly with neurological disorders undergoing enteral nutrition therapy. *Rev. Assoc. Med. Bras.* **2012**, *58*, 691–697. [CrossRef] [PubMed]

31. Kumagai, R.; Kubokura, M.; Sano, A.; Shinomiya, M.; Ohta, S.; Ishibiki, Y.; Narumi, K.; Aiba, M.; Ichimiya, Y. Clinical evaluation of percutaneous endoscopic gastrostomy tube feeding in Japanese patients with dementia. *Psychiatry Clin. Neurosci.* **2012**, *66*, 418–422. [CrossRef] [PubMed]

32. Blomberg, J.; Lagergren, P.; Martin, L.; Mattsson, F.; Lagergren, J. Albumin and C-reactive protein levels predict short-term mortality after percutaneous endoscopic gastrostomy in a prospective cohort study. *Gastrointest. Endosc.* **2011**, *73*, 29–36. [CrossRef] [PubMed]

33. Schneider, A.S.; Schettler, A.; Markowski, A.; Luettig, B.; Kaufmann, B.; Klamt, S.; Lenzen, H.; Momma, M.; Seipt, C.; Lankisch, T.; *et al.* Complication and mortality rate after percutaneous endoscopic gastrostomy are low and indication-dependent. *Scand. J. Gastroenterol.* **2014**, *49*, 891–898. [CrossRef] [PubMed]

34. Goel, M.K.; Khanna, P.; Kishorel, J. Understanding survival analysis: Kaplan-Meier estimate. *Int. J. Ayurveda Res.* **2010**, *1*, 274–278. [CrossRef] [PubMed]

35. Mitchell, S.L.; Kiely, D.K.; Lipstiz, L.A. The risk factors and impact on survival of feeding tube placement in nursing home and residents with severe cognitive impairment. *Arch. Intern. Med.* **1997**, *157*, 327–332. [CrossRef] [PubMed]

36. Meier, D.E.; Ahronheim, J.C.; Morris, J.; Baskin-Lyons, S.; Morrison, R.S. High short-term mortality in hospitalized patients with advanced dementia. Lack of benefit of tube feeding. *Arch. Intern. Med.* **2001**, *161*, 594–599. [CrossRef] [PubMed]

37. Goldberg, L.S.; Althman, K.W. The role of gastrostomy tube placement in advanced dementia with dysphagia: A critical review. *Clin. Interv. Aging* **2014**, *9*, 1733–1739. [CrossRef] [PubMed]

38. Murtagh, F.E.M.; Preston, M.; Higginson, I. Patterns of dying: Palliative care for non-malignant disease. *Clin. Med.* **2004**, *4*, 39–44. [CrossRef] [PubMed]

39. Murray, S.A.; Kendall, M.; Boyd, K.; Sheikh, A. Illness trajectories and palliative care. *BMJ* **2005**, *330*, 1007–1011. [CrossRef] [PubMed]

40. Janes, S.E.; Price, C.S.; Khan, S. Percutaneous endoscopic gastrostomy: 30 day mortality trends and risk factors. *J. Post. Grad. Med.* **2005**, *51*, 23–29.

41. Lang, A.; Bardan, E.; Chowers, Y.; Sakhnini, E.; Fidder, H.H.; Bar-Meir, S.; Avidan, B. Risk factors for mortality in patients undergoing percutaneous endoscopic gastrostomy. *Endoscopy* **2004**, *36*, 522–526. [CrossRef] [PubMed]

42. Shah, P.M.; Sen, S.; Perlmuter, L.C.; Feller, A. Survival after percutaneous endoscopic gastrostomy: The role of dementia. *J. Nutr. Health Aging* **2005**, *9*, 255–259. [PubMed]

43. Nicholson, J.P.; Wolmarans, M.R.; Park, G.R. The role of albumin in critical illness. *Brit. J. Anaesth.* **2000**, *85*, 599–610. [CrossRef] [PubMed]

44. Klonoff-Cohen, H.; Barrett-Connor, E.L.; Edelstein, S.L. Albumin levels as a predictor of mortality in the healthy elderly. *J. Clin. Epidemiol.* **1992**, *45*, 207–212. [CrossRef] [PubMed]

45. Terekeci, H.; Kucukardali, Y.; Top, C.; Onem, Y.; Celik, S.; Oktenli, C. Risk assessment study of pressure ulcers in intensive care unit patients. *Eur. J. Intern. Med.* **2009**, *20*, 394–397. [CrossRef] [PubMed]

46. Ho, C.H.; Powell, H.I.; Collins, J.F.; Bauman, W.A.; Spunquen, A.M. Poor nutrition is a relative contraindication for negative pressure wound therapy for pressure uclers: Preliminary observations in patients with spinal cord injury. *Adv. Skin Wound Care* **2010**, *23*, 508–516. [CrossRef] [PubMed]

47. Suzaki, Y. Enteral Nutrition—PEG indiction. *Nihon Ishikai Zasshi* **2009**, *138*, 1767–1770.

48. Korner, U.; Bondolfi, A.; Buhler, E.; MacFie, J.; Meguid, M.M.; Messing, B.; Oehmichen, F.; Valentini, L.; Allison, A.P. Ethical and legal aspects of Enteral Nutrition. *Clin. Nutr.* **2006**, *25*, 196–200. [CrossRef] [PubMed]

49. Downs, M.; Mackenzie, J.; Clare, L. Understanding of dementia: Explanatory models and their implications for the person with dementia and their therapeutic effort. In *Dementia, Mind, Meaning and Person*; Hughes, J.C., Louw, S.J., Sabat, S.R., Eds.; Oxford University Press: Oxford, UK, 2006.

50. Banerjee, S.; Smith, S.C.; Lamping, D.L.; Harwood, R.H.; Foley, B.; Smith, P.; Murray, J.; Prince, M.; Levin, E.; Mann, A.; *et al.* Quality of life in dementia: More than just cognition. An analysis of association with quality of life in dementia. *Neurol. Neurosurg. Psychiatry* **2006**, *77*, 146–148. [CrossRef]

51. Royal College of Physicians and British Society of Gastroenterology. Oral Feeding Difficulties and Dilemmas. A Guide to Practical Care, Particularly towards End of Life. 2010. Available online: https://www.rcplondon. ac.uk/sites/default/files/documents/oral-feeding-difficulties-and-dilemmas.pdf (assessed on 1 July 2014).

52. Rabeneck, L.; McCullough, L.B.; Wray, N.P. Ethically justified, clinically comprehensive guidelines for percutaneous endoscopic gastrostomy tube placement. *Lancet* **1997**, *349*, 496–498. [CrossRef] [PubMed]

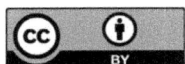

nutrients

MDPI

Review

The Challenges of Home Enteral Tube Feeding: A Global Perspective

Omorogieva Ojo

Faculty of Education and Health,University of Greenwich, Avery Hill Campus, Avery Hill Road, London SE9 2UG, UK; o.ojo@greenwich.ac.uk; Tel.: +44-(0)20-8331-8626; Fax: +44(0)20-8331-8060

Received: 16 December 2014; Accepted: 1 April 2015; Published: 8 April 2015

Abstract: The aim of this review is to provide a global perspective of Home Enteral Tube Feeding (HETF) and to outline some of the challenges of home enteral nutrition (HEN) provisions. It is well established that the number of patients on HETF is on the increase worldwide due to advances in technology, development of percutaneous endoscopic gastrostomy techniques, and the shift in care provisions from acute to community settings. While the significance of home enteral nutrition in meeting the nutritional requirements of patients with poor swallowing reflexes and those with poor nutritional status is not in doubt, differences exist in terms of funding, standards, management approaches and the level of infrastructural development across the world. Strategies for alleviating some of the challenges militating against the effective delivery of HETF including the development of national and international standards, guidelines and policies for HETF, increased awareness and funding by government at all levels were discussed. Others, including development of HEN services, which should create the enabling environment for multidisciplinary team work, clinical audit and research, recruitment and retention of specialist staff, and improvement in patient outcomes have been outlined. However, more research is required to fully establish the cost effectiveness of the HEN service especially in developing countries and to compare the organization of HEN service between developing and developed countries.

Keywords: enteral tube feeding; community; global perspective; developing countries; developed countries; home enteral nutrition

1. Introduction

This article aims to provide an overview of the worldwide perspective of home enteral tube feeding (HETF) and outline some of the challenges of home enteral nutrition (HEN) provisions. Enteral tube feeding is an effective method of providing nutrients for individuals who are unable to meet their nutritional requirements in different healthcare settings across the world [1–3]. In a study by Klek *et al.* [4] in Poland, implementation of HEN improved clinical outcomes and decreased health care costs through weight gain in patients, reduced incidence of infectious complications and the number of hospital admissions. In another study in Malawi, Brewster *et al.* [5] reported that routine tube-feeding was associated with improved body weight gain in the treatment of kwashiorkor (protein deficiency). A nutritional support team in Nigeria has used high calorie enteral feed in the management of protein energy malnutrition in children [6]. On the other hand, HEN has been shown to improve the nutritional status and quality of life in patients with advanced gastric cancer in China [7].

The use of HETF has become more common globally due to advances in technology, development of percutaneous endoscopic gastrostomy (PEG) technique and governments' policy of shifting healthcare provisions from costly acute hospitals to community settings [8–11]. These have also ensured that more individuals on enteral feeds now live in the community. In the UK, a 42.78% increase over a 10-year period in patients receiving HEN has been reported [12], although there is evidence of a yearly increase (20%–25%) in the number of people on enteral feed [13]. According to Moreno Villares [14], home enteral nutrition was developed after home parenteral nutrition, however, it has grown rapidly in some countries. There are significant international differences in prevalence and growth rate of home enteral nutrition, in the organisation of nutritional support services, and in financial arrangements [15]. Although the incidence of HETF may be difficult to determine, estimates of 460 (United States) and 40 (Spain) patients per million inhabitants have been reported [14]. In most countries around the world, neurological diseases, such as cerebrovascular accident, multiple sclerosis, and cancer especially, head and neck cancer, are the most frequent indications for HETF [12,14].

In a previous study by Ojo [12] in the UK, 187 out of the 257 patients on HETF, representing 72.76% were receiving enteral nutrition through percutaneous endoscopic gastrostomy. This value appears similar in other parts of Europe, although this only occurs in 25% of cases in Spain [14].

Despite worldwide application of HETF, significant differences remain between developed and developing countries in terms of the challenges, especially with respect to funding, organisation, infrastructure, procurement of feeds, pump, ancillary items, research and development, and management of patients and related complications.

Organisation of Home Enteral Tube Feeding

Irrespective of the strategy for delivering HEN service, the procurement and supply of enteral feeding pump, feed and ancillary items require an effective process in order to ensure a seamless delivery and promotion of patients' outcomes. This is essential because there should be continuity of service provision and enteral nutrition management when patients are discharged home from hospital. In the USA and UK, national standards require patients on HETF to be well trained, to have written protocols for trouble-shooting and for undertaking routine procedures, and to have 24-h telephone contacts in cases of emergency. While these have been developed in the US and UK, other countries appear to have local standards [15].

Furthermore, in the USA, the role of companies in the supply and delivery of pumps, feed, ancillary items, management of patients on HEN and associated complications is quite significant while in Europe, HEN is usually coordinated from regional or district hospitals [15]. Other approaches to HEN in the USA have been outlined by Newton and Barnadas [3], who reported that home enteral nutrition is often started without the usual resources of the hospital. In addition, dieticians working in home care mostly assume primary role in patient care and management, and have to have knowledge and expertise with the wide variety of enteral equipment and access devices.

In Poland, there is evidence that HEN includes complex monitoring by a nutrition support team [4]. With respect to the UK, enteral feed, feeding accessories and pump are supplied to patients in the community through different strategies and the management could be one or a combination of the following; self care, carers, care home registered nurses, general practitioner (GP), Home enteral feeding service provided by a dietician, community nursing service, Home care company and the HEN team [16].

However, two of the most common methods of supplying patients with enteral feed, feeding accessories and pump in the UK are Hospital Enteral Nutrition Service and Community or Home Enteral Nutrition (HEN) Service.

Under the Hospital Enteral Nutrition service, the nutrition department or the nutrition team based in hospital is responsible for the care and management of patients on HEN including the supply of feed, feeding accessories and pump in hospital and home. The nutrition support team in hospital often provides home visits or outpatient clinics and for those patients who have been discharged home from hospital, the continued supply of feed and feeding accessories is usually by means of prescription using the FP10 (prescription form) [16,17]. The delivery of the feeding pumps to HEN patients is often through the community nursing. National Health Service (NHS) supplies organisations, or the receive the equipment directly from the manufacturer and costs are charged back to the hospital budget [18].

In contrast, the UK Community or Home Enteral Nutrition Service is usually multidisciplinary team that consists of healthcare professionals and support staff who have diverse clinical qualifications, skills, knowledge and experience [19]. These specialist healthcare professionals include the nutrition nurse specialist, dietician, and speech and language therapist. One of the primary features of the HEN service is that patients' feeds are managed "off script" and therefore do not require the use of FP10 [20]. The HEN service is the model of choice and requires a clear pathway between acute and community care and other partners including companies in order to ensure an effective delivery system [8,21,22]. In a study that compared hospital enteral nutrition and home enteral nutrition in China, Wang *et al.* [23] reported that patients with intestinal fistulae in the HEN group had shorter hospital stay than patients in the hospital group. Furthermore, the cost of treatment was significantly lower and the quality of life significantly improved in the HEN group compared with the Hospital enteral nutrition group. In studies from a number of countries around the world reviewed by Majka *et al.* [24], multiple intervention strategies were adopted in the management of enteral tube feeding.

Based on the above, the objective of this review is as follows;

- To explore the issues around home enteral tube feeding in providing nutritional support globally.

The research question is:

- Are there challenges in the use of home enteral tube feeding as a global strategy in nutritional support provision?

2. Method

This review involved a literature search of articles on challenges of home enteral nutrition across the globe. It included a general scoping of the databases, which found one systematic review on international perspective on artificial nutritional support in the community published in 1995 by Elia [15]. This review based its findings on evidence drawn from studies relating to both Home parenteral and enteral nutrition. Since the publication, a number of other studies have been published which form the basis for the current review.

The main data bases searched included EBSCO Host/Health Sciences Research databases (encompassing Academic search premier, Medline, Psychology and Behavioural sciences collection, PSYCINFO, SPORTDISCUSS and Cumulative Index to Nursing and Allied Literature (CINAHL) Plus, PubMed and SwetsWise. The search terms included; challenges of enteral nutrition, challenges "and" home enteral tube feeding, enteral nutrition "and" Europe, enteral nutrition "and" Africa, enteral nutrition "and" South America, enteral nutrition "and" Asia, enteral nutrition "and" central America, enteral nutrition "and" America, enteral nutrition "and" Australia.

2.1. Inclusion and Exclusion Criteria

Searches included articles published between 1995 and 2014 covering the areas of interest except, one study that was published in 1988 and was included due to the limited studies published on Africa. Only studies written in English language were included and those that did not meet the above inclusion criteria were excluded from the current review.

2.2. Data Analysis

Based on the criteria outlined for exclusion and inclusion, eight studies on enteral nutrition complications (Table 1) were selected. Seven studies on cost effectiveness of enteral nutrition (Table 2) were also included although some of these studies were previously cited in Table 1. Most of these studies were conducted in Europe, North America and Australia. While studies carried out in developing countries in these aspects of enteral nutrition were limited, there were studies from around the world that provided an overview of the challenges of enteral nutrition, which were included.

3. Results

With respect to enteral nutrition complications, the results show that across the globe, the main sources of enteral nutrition complications are due to stoma site infection, tube dislodgement, tube blockage, tube leakage, diarrhoea, overgranulation, vomiting, and pneumonia (Table 1).

While formation of overgranulation tissue (67%) was the highest form of complication in Canada [25], constipation (48%) was the highest in Ireland [26]. In Greece, inadvertent removal of tube (45.1%) was highest and in Australia insertion site infection was 41% [27,28]. In Turkey, while tube displacement was highest at 7.6%, wound infection was 3.3% [29]. Overgranulation of PEG site was 26.7% compared with 6.7% for balloon gastrostomy site in the UK, while pneumonia was the most frequent form of complication at 55.9% in Brazil [1,30].

With respect to the findings on the cost effectiveness of enteral nutrition, one study showed variation in the daily overall costs of HEN from 7 to 25 Euros across Europe [31] (Table 2). On the other hand, studies in Poland and the US showed significant improvements in patient outcomes and cost of hospitalisation following implementation of HEN and nutrition support clinic [4,32]

One study in the US revealed that HEN is significantly cheaper compared with Home parenteral nutrition [33]. The Australian study showed that inpatient cost of PEG patients was significantly more than for patients on nasogastric feeding tube (NGT) [28]. The UK study found that the cost effectiveness of enteral tube feeding, where non-medical costs are paid privately, compares favourably with other interventions, but it was not so when the state pays all non-medical costs [34]. The study which compared the impact of home and hospital enteral nutrition in China found that the HEN group had shorter hospital stay, significant reduction in cost of treatment, improved quality of life although no significant difference in the incidence of complications [23].

4. Discussion

4.1. Challenges of Current Organisation of Home Enteral Tube Feeding

In developed countries of Europe and the USA, where organised HEN services exist, challenges in the areas of funding, the number of HEN services, research and development, multidisciplinary team working, managing the HEN service including problems with delivering enteral feed and accessories and complications due to pump, feed and stoma site are often the main issues of concern [1,12,27,32, 35,36]. Details of these difficulties of the HEN service globally have been fully outlined in Table 1. For example, in the UK, many National Health Service (NHS) Trusts do not have a HEN team and this will limit their capacity for service improvement and delivery [19].

Funding is a major challenge in the management of HETF anywhere in the world and with the on-going economic crisis influencing health care, its cost-effectiveness has been questioned [4]. British Artificial Nutrition Survey (BANS) reports that 40% of centres have no budget allocated specifically for enteral nutrition support [10].

According to Elia [15], the use of home enteral nutrition in different countries appears to be generally related to the overall expenditure on health (government and private), and percentage of the gross domestic product (GDP) expended on health. In Asian countries such as India and Pakistan, and in many parts of Africa, where the figure is less than 4%–5% of the GDP, home enteral nutrition is not common [15]. By contrast, in the USA where the GDP expended on health from private expenditure alone was 11.7% in 1991, home enteral nutrition is used more than anywhere else in the world [15]. This is followed closely by Western European countries where expenditure on health is usually 6%–9% of GDP although estimates from eastern European countries with limited information is likely to be low [15]. For example, in the UK based hospital enteral nutrition service, the effective management of feed, pump and ancillary items, and patients on HEN may be affected because there is no dedicated team in the community to follow up in the care and maintenance of the service. Under this method, the unit cost of feed is much higher because individual patient in the community rely on the use of FP10 (prescription form) to procure their feed compared to when feeds and feeding accessories are purchased in larger quantities [18]. In addition, due to conflicting pressures dietetic support may not be routinely available for patients on HETF, even on outpatient basis.

Although the community home enteral nutrition service purchases feed "off script" and thus can save money from the bulk purchase of feeds, challenge of multidisciplinary team working can militate against effective service delivery. For example, although the roles and responsibilities of the different HCPs are distinct, there are areas of overlap, which may become sources of friction. The number of different HCPs working within the HEN team who visit the patients regularly for assessment and reviews can become blurry and confusing to the patients due to their number and different times of visits [19].

Due to the specialist nature of the HEN service, recruitment and retention of qualified staff are some of the difficulties providers have to address. Therefore, it is not uncommon to find some HEN services having developmental roles such as Nutrition Support Nurse, Nutrition Nurse Specialist working alongside the Clinical Lead Nutrition Nurse Specialist [8].

Despite the worldwide recognition of HETF as a useful method of meeting the nutritional requirements of patients and as a life-saving procedure, difficulties often arise during and post tube insertion. These problems appear to the similar globally although the levels of prevalence may vary [25,26,28–30,37] (Table 1).

Other possible challenges confronting the HEN service include the supply of feed, pump and ancillary items. Evans *et al.* [38] reported that 20% of patients receiving HEN were not contacted until seven days or more after discharge in the UK. In addition, 47% of patients did not receive a delivery until seven or more days after discharge, while 41% reported missing equipment from their first delivery. In the same study, 17% of patients reported difficulty getting their GP to write a prescription. Those patients whose deliveries were not organised directly with the home delivery company by the hospital were more likely to have delayed delivery of seven or more days after discharge (63% compared with 21% of those directly organised by regional hospital) [38].

Table 1. Incidence of Enteral Feeding Complications.

Citation	Country of Study	Type of Study	Number of Patients	Outcomes
Hall et al., 2014 [32]	USA	Retrospective quality analysis	52 patients	- Approximately 30% of patients seen at least once for clogged tube and 43.3% for tube leakage. - One patient required a procedure for tube re-insertion
Corry et al., 2009 [28]	Australia	Prospective study to compare PEG tubes and NGT tubes in terms of nutritional outcomes	32 PEG and 73 nasogastric tube (NGT) patients	- PEG patients had significantly less weight loss at 6 weeks post treatment (median 0.8 kg gain *versus* 3.7 kg loss), but had a higher insertion site infection rate (41%). - There was 62% tube dislodgement in the NGT group compared with 19% for PEG group
Alivizatos et al., 2012 [27]	Greece	Retrospective review of medical records	31	Accidental removal of tube (broken tube, plugged tube; 45.1%), tube leakage (6.4%), dermatitis of the stoma (6.4%), diarrhoea (6.4%)
McNamara et al., 2000 [26]	Ireland	Retrospective survey	50	Blocked tube (30%), local infection at stoma site (16%), tube replacement (26%), diarrhoea (34%), vomiting (40%), constipation (48%)
Crosby and Duerksen, 2005 [25]	Canada	Retrospective Survey	55 out of 221 patients completed the survey	Granulation tissue formation (67%), broken or leaking tube (56%), leakage around the tube site (60%), stoma infection requiring antibiotics (45%)
Martins et al., 2012 [30]	Brazil	-	79 patients	- 91.2% presented some complications such as pneumonia, catheter loss, diarrhoea, constipation, fluid leakage, tube obstruction, reflux. - Pneumonia was the most frequent complication, occurring in 55.9% of cases
Ojo, 2011 [1]	UK	Retrospective review	30 patients	Overgranulation of stoma site (PEG, 26.7%; Balloon gastrostomy tube, 6.7%; infected stoma site (PEG, 6.7%; Balloon gastrostomy tube, 13.3%) during initial visit.
Erdil et al., 2005 [29]	Turkey	-	85 patients	More than 30 days after insertion of PEG; Tube occlusion (4.3%), tube displacement (7.6%), wound infection (3.3%), peristomal leakage (2.2%), reflux and vomiting (1.1%), peritonitis (1.1%).

Table 2. The Cost—effectiveness of Enteral Nutrition.

Citation	Country of Study	Type of Study	Number of Patients	Outcomes
Klek et al., 2014 [4]	Poland	Observational multicentre study	456 HEN patients	- HEN enabled weight gain, stabilised liver function. - HEN implementation reduced incidence of infectious complications (37.4% compared with 14.9%), the number of hospital admissions [1.98 ± 2.42 (mean ± SD)] before and 1.26 ± 2.18 after enteral nutrition. - The length of hospital stay was 39.7 ± 71.9 compared with 11.9 ± 28.8 days. - The mean annual costs ($) of hospitalisation were reduced from 6500.20 ± 10,402.69 to 2072.58 ± 5497.00
Reddy, 1998 [33]	USA	Retrospective Review	-	For Home parenteral and Home enteral nutrition respectively: Annual cost per patient solution ($55,193 ± 30,596; 9605 ± 9327) (mean ± SD), annual cost of hospitalisation (0–$140,220; 0–$39,204), Annual number of hospitalisations per patient (0.52–1.10; 0–0.5). Health status (significantly lower; significantly higher).
Hall et al., 2014 [32]	USA	A retrospective quality analysis	52 patients	Complications and high cost interventions, including emergency room visits, hospital admissions and surgical tube re-insertions were significantly reduced after implementation of nutrition support clinic.
Elia and Stratton, 2008 [34]	UK	Cost-utility analysis	-	- The cost effectiveness of enteral tube feeding in patients with cerebral vascular accident receiving enteral tube feeding at home or nursing homes, where the non-medical costs are paid privately compared favourably with other interventions. - The cost effectiveness of enteral tube feeding in nursing homes when the state pays all non-medical costs compared unfavourably with other treatments.
Corry et al., 2009 [28]	Australia	Prospective study to compare PEG tubes and NGT tubes in terms of nutritional outcomes	32 PEG and 73 NGT patients	- The median nights stay in hospital was 4 for the NGT patients compared with 14 for the PEG patients. - The inpatient cost for PEG patients would be $3556 versus $1016 (Australian dollars) for the NGT group.
Wang et al., 2013 [23]	China	Comparative study between Home enteral nutrition and Hospital enteral nutrition	Home enteral nutrition =42; Hospital enteral nutrition = 40; Normal control = 40	- The HEN group had shorter hospital stay, significant reduction in cost of treatment and improved quality of life. - No significant difference in the incidence of complications
Hebuterne et al., 2003 [31]	Belgium, Denmark, France, Germany, Italy, Poland, Spain, UK	A European Multicentre Survey	1397	- Daily costs of HEN were not available in centres from Denmark and the UK. - In other centres of Europe, the daily overall costs of HEN varied from 7 to 25 Euros. - These costs include costs of the formula, the infusion pump, micronutrients, bags, tubing and dressing and do not include cost of the care giver, cost of re-hospitalisation and medical monitoring.

4.2. Cost Effectiveness of Home Enteral Nutrition

The cost effectiveness of home enteral nutrition may be assessed based on the service being provided and strategies for delivering the service [28,31,32,34]. Details of the cost-effectiveness of the HEN service are clearly outlined in Table 2. In a systematic review and meta-analysis of studies across the world, Majka *et al.* [24] showed that 93.3% of the studies reviewed reported beneficial effects in terms of patients' outcomes, staff outcomes and costs of care due to care coordination and/or team approach. These views are related to the findings of the current review which show that the HEN service provide significant improvement in patients' outcomes [4,23,33].

Patient outcomes may be based on mortality, quality of life scores, infections and hospital admissions [28,31,32,34]. According to Majka *et al.* [24], the average hospital cost per patient was reduced by $623.08. In another review conducted by Michael *et al.* [39] in the USA, it was reported that the average savings from enteral nutrition due to reduced adverse event risks was about $1500 per patient and savings from reduced hospital length of stay was about $2500 per patient. It was noted that shifting 10% of adult patients in the USA managed parenterally to enteral nutrition would save $35 million annually due to reduced adverse events and another $57 million from shorter stays in hospital [39].

Pritchard *et al.* [40] reported that observational non-randomised studies that compared groups receiving parenteral and enteral nutrition found few differences in clinical outcomes between groups but showed lower costs in enteral nutrition patients. For example, while in 19 US patients about to have major abdominal surgery, mean daily costs for enteral nutrition were just under half the costs of parenteral nutrition of about $100 pay, in 24 UK patients undergoing orthotopic liver transplantation, there was a 10-fold difference (£7 per day compared with £75–85) [40].

Wilhelm *et al.* [41] carried out a theoretical cost analysis between inpatients and outpatients on percutaneous endoscopic gastrostomy in the US. According to the authors, the actual outpatient charge was $135 per patient compared to $1155 per patient for a theoretical admission. A potential cost savings of $29,120 in 26 out-patient procedures and a projected average cost savings per patient of $1020 were reported by Wilhelm *et al.* [41].

5. Strategies for Improving Home Enteral Tube Feeding

There is urgent need to develop the infrastructure for HEN service in developing countries in Africa, Asia and South America in order to meet the needs of the patients who may require these services. With respect to developed countries of Europe and North America, there is the need to improve cooperation and communication between nurses in hospitals and in communities, as well as for increasing nurses' level of knowledge, to make home enteral tube feeding work in a safe way [42]. In addition, the roles and responsibilities should be clarified between the different healthcare professionals who should also understand guidelines for the care of tube feeding and discharge process [43–45]. There should also be clear pathways of referral and communication between acute, community, companies and patients.

The establishment of national regulations and legislation (or even regional regulations within a country) should be encouraged because they provide important advantages, including a uniform distribution of specialist HEN services across the country and clear financial guidelines, which should ensure that appropriate standards for selection and management are attained ensuring that government departments are fully aware of the issues involved [15].

In addition, it is essential to build trust between the different professions in the team, and support colleagues to take on new roles that are not normally associated with their traditional roles [26,46]. As part of the building of effective multidisciplinary HEN team, it will be useful to have regular training, away days, caseload review meetings and a team charter in place.

Creating the enabling environment for HCPs working within the HEN service to conduct research and clinical audits will no doubt provide the opportunity for service improvement and staff development. The issue of inappropriate placements of enteral feeding tubes and/or overprescription of enteral feed and ancillary items could have far reaching implications in terms of costs to the health service. A useful strategy could be to ensure appropriateness of indications of enteral nutrition provisions and the range of feeding tubes and accessories.

6. Conclusions

Home enteral tube feeding is a useful method of supporting the nutritional needs of patients in the community who are unable to meet their nutritional requirements through oral intake alone. Although its use has been globally acclaimed, differences exist in home enteral nutrition provisions across the world.

The factors militating against the effective delivery of HEN service include; funding, level of organisation, lack of national and international standards and infrastructure, problems of procurement of feeds, pump, ancillary items, research and development, and management of patients and associated complications including tube and stoma complications.

In order to address these problems, there has to be development of national and international standards, guidelines and policies for enteral nutrition provisions, increased awareness and funding by government at all levels, development of HEN services that will provide the enabling environment for multidisciplinary team work, clinical audit and research, recruitment and retention of specialist staff, and improvement in patient outcomes. However, more research is needed to fully establish the cost effectiveness of the HEN service especially in developing countries and to compare the prevalence of complications, cost implications and organization between developed and developing countries.

Conflicts of Interest: The author declares no conflict of interest.

References

1. Ojo, O. Balloon gastrostomy tubes for long-term feeding in the community. *Br. J. Nurs.* **2011**, *20*, 34–38. [CrossRef] [PubMed]
2. Fogg, L. Home enteral feeding Part 1: An overview. *Br. J. Nurs.* **2007**, *12*, 246–252. [CrossRef]
3. Rowat, A. Enteral tube feeding for dysphagic stroke patients. *Br. J. Nurs.* **2015**, *24*, 138–145. [CrossRef] [PubMed]
4. Klek, S.; Hermanowicz, A.; Dziwiszek, G.; Matysiak, K.; Szczepanek, K.; Szybinski, P.; Galas, A. Home enteral nutrition reduces complications, length of stay, and health care costs: Results from a multicenter study. *Am. J. Clin. Nutr.* **2014**, *100*, 609–615. [CrossRef] [PubMed]
5. Brewster, D.R.; Manary, M.J.; Graham, S.M. Case management of kwashiorkor: An intervention project at seven nutrition rehabilitation centres in Malawi. *Eur. J. Clin. Nutr.* **1997**, *51*, 139–147. [CrossRef] [PubMed]
6. Ojofeitimi, E.O.; Smith, I.F. Nutrition support and malnutrition in Nigeria. *Nutr. Clin. Pract.* **1988**, *3*, 242–245. [CrossRef] [PubMed]
7. Qian, Z.; Sun, Y.; Ye, Z.; Shao, Q.; Xu, X. Application of home enteral nutrition and its impact on the quality of life in patients with advanced gastric cancer. *Chin. J. Gastrointest. Surg.* **2014**, *17*, 158–162.
8. Ojo, O. The impact of changes in health and social care on enteral feeding in the community. *Nutrients* **2012**, *4*, 1709–1722. [CrossRef] [PubMed]
9. Department of Health. *Shifting Care Closer to Home Care Closer to Home Demonstration Sites—Report of the Speciality Subgroups*; Department of Health: London, UK, 2007.
10. Madigan, S.M.; O'Neill, S.; Clarke, J.; L'Estrange, F.; MacAuley, D.C. Assessing the dietetic needs of different patient groups receiving enteral tube feeding in primary care. *J. Hum. Nutr. Diet.* **2002**, *15*, 179–184. [CrossRef] [PubMed]
11. NHS Institute for Innovation and Improvement. *Making the Shift: Key Success Factors a Rapid Review of Best Practice in Shifting Hospital Care into the Community*; HSMC: London, UK, 2006.
12. Ojo, O. Managing patients on enteral feeding tubes in the community. *Br. J. Community Nurs.* **2010**, *15*, S6–S13.
13. Russell, C.A. Home enteral tube feeding: The role of the industry. *Clin. Nutr.* **2001**, *20* (Suppl. 1), 67–69. [CrossRef]

14. Moreno Villares, J.M. The practice of home artificial nutrition in Europe. *Nutr. Hosp.* **2004**, *19*, 59–67. [PubMed]

15. Elia, M. An international perspective on artificial nutritional support in the community. *Lancet* **1995**, *345*, 1345–1349. [CrossRef] [PubMed]

16. Green, S.; Dinenage, S.; Gower, M.; van Wyk, J. Home enteral nutrition: Organisation of services. *Nurs. Older People* **2013**, *25*, 14–18. [CrossRef] [PubMed]

17. Joint Formulary Committee. *British National Formulary 66*; BMJ Group and Pharmaceutical Press: London, UK, 2013.

18. Howard, P.; Bowen, N. The challenges of innovation in the organization of home enteral tube feeding. *J. Hum. Nutr. Diet.* **2001**, *14*, 3–11. [CrossRef] [PubMed]

19. Ojo, O.; Patel, I. Home enteral nutrition and team working. *J. Community Nurs.* **2012**, *26*, 15–18.

20. Best, C.; Hitchings, H. Enteral tube feeding—From hospital to home. *Br. J. Nurs.* **2010**, *19*, 174–179. [CrossRef] [PubMed]

21. Jones, A. Multidisciplinary team working: Collaboration and conflict. *Int. J. Ment. Health Nurs.* **2006**, *15*, 19–28. [CrossRef] [PubMed]

22. Nicholson, D.; Artz, S.; Armitage, A.; Fagan, J. Working relationships and outcomes in multidisciplinary collaborative practice settings. *Child Youth Care Forum.* **2000**, *29*, 39–73. [CrossRef]

23. Wang, Y.; Kang, Y.; Zhou, J.R. Comparison of two types of enteral nutrition in patients with intestinal fistula. *Zhonghua Yi Xue Za Zhi* **2013**, *93*, 2364–2366.

24. Majka, A.J.; Wang, Z.; Schmitz, K.R.; Niesen, C.R.; Larsen, R.A.; Kinsey, G.C.; Murad, A.L.; Prokop, L.J.; Murad, M.H. Care coordination to enhance management of long-term enteral tube feeding: a systematic review and meta-analysis. *J. Parenter. Enter. Nutr.* **2014**, *38*, 40–52. [CrossRef]

25. Crosby, J.; Duerksen, D. A retrospective survey of tube-related complications in patients receiving long-term home enteral nutrition. *Dig. Dis. Sci.* **2005**, *50*, 1712–1717. [CrossRef] [PubMed]

26. McNamara, E.P.; Flood, P.; Kennedy, N.P. Enteral tube feeding in the community: Survey of adult patients discharged from a Dublin hospital. *Clin. Nutr.* **2000**, *19*, 15–22. [CrossRef] [PubMed]

27. Alivizatos, V.; Gavala, V.; Alexopoulos, P.; Apostolopoulos, A.; Bajrucevic, S. Feeding Tube-related Complications and Problems in Patients Receiving Long-term Home Enteral Nutrition. *Indian J. Palliat. Care* **2012**, *18*, 31–33. [CrossRef] [PubMed]

28. Corry, J.; Poon, W.; Mcphee, N.; Milner, A.D.; Cruickshank, D.; Porceddu, S.V.; Rixchin, D.; Peters, L.J. Prospective study of percutaneous endoscopic gastrostomy tubes *versus* nasogastric tubes for enteral feeding in patients with head and neck cancer undergoing (chemo) radiation. *Head Neck* **2009**, *31*, 867–876. [CrossRef] [PubMed]

29. Erdil, A.; Saka, M.; Ates, Y.; Tuzun, A.; Bagci, S.; Uygun, A.; Zeki, Y.; Gulsen, M.; Karaeren, N.; Dagalp, K. Enteral nutrition via percutaneous endoscopic gastrostomy and nutritional status of patients: Five-year prospective study. *J. Gastroenterol. Hepatol.* **2005**, *20*, 1002–1007. [CrossRef]

30. Martins, A.S; Rezende, N.A.; Torres, H.O. Occurrence of complications and survival rates in elderly with neurological disorders undergoing enteral nutrition therapy. *Rev. Assoc. Med. Bras.* **2012**, *58*, 691–697. [CrossRef]

31. Hebuterne, X.; Bozzetti, F.; Moreno Villares, J.M.; Pertkiewicz, M.; Shaffer, J.; Staun, M.; Thul, P.; van Gossum, A. ESPEN—Home Artificial Nutrition working Group. *Clin. Nutr.* **2003**, *22*, 261–266. [CrossRef] [PubMed]

32. Hall, B.T.; Englehart, M.S.; Blaseg, K.; Wessel, K.; Stawicki, S.P.A.; Evans, D.C. Implementation of a dietitian-led enteral nutrition support clinic results in quality improvement, reduced readmissions, and cost savings. *Nutr. Clin. Pract.* **2014**, *29*, 649–655. [CrossRef]

33. Reddy, P. Cost and outcome analysis of home parenteral and enteral nutrition. *J. Parenter. Enter. Nutr.* **1998**, *22*, 302–310. [CrossRef]

34. Elia, M.; Stratton, R.J. A cost-utility analysis in patients receiving enteral tube feeding at home and in nursing homes. *Clin. Nutr.* **2008**, *27*, 416–423. [CrossRef] [PubMed]

35. Ojo, O.; Bowden, J. Infection control in enteral feed and feeding systems in the community. *Br. J. Nurs.* **2012**, *21*, 1070–1075. [CrossRef]

36. Ojo, O. Problems with use of a Foley catheter in home enteral tube feeding. *Br. J. Nurs.* **2014**, *23*, 360–364. [CrossRef] [PubMed]

37. Ojo, O. Evaluating Care: Home enteral nutrition. *J. Community Nurs.* **2010**, *24*, 18–25.

38. Evans, S.; MacDonald, A.; Holden, C. Home enteral feeding audit. *J. Hum. Nutr. Diet.* **2004**, *17*, 537–542. [CrossRef]

39. Michael, J.C.; Hannah, R.A.; Joshua, T.C. A clinical and economic evaluation of enteral nutrition. *Curr. Med. Res. Opin.* **2011**, *27*, 413–422. [CrossRef] [PubMed]

40. Pritchard, C.; Duffy, S.; Edington, J.; Pang, F. Enteral nutrition and oral nutrition supplements: A review of the economics literature. *J. Parenter. Enter. Nutr.* **2006**, *30*, 52–59. [CrossRef]

41. Wilhelm, S.M.; Ortega, K.A.; Stellato, T.A. Guidelines for identification and management of outpatient percutaneous endoscopic gastrostomy tube placement. *Am. J. Surg.* **2010**, *199*, 396–400. [CrossRef] [PubMed]

42. Bjuresater, K.; Larsson, M.; Nord Strom, G.; Athlin, E. Cooperation in the care for patients with home enteral tube throughout the care trajectory: Nurses perspectives. *J. Clin. Nurs.* **2008**, *17*, 3021–3029. [CrossRef] [PubMed]

43. Doyle, J. Barriers and facilitators of multidisciplinary team working: A review. *Paediatr. Nurs.* **2008**, *20*, 26–29. [PubMed]

44. Hansson, A.; Friberg, F.; Segesten, K.; Gedda, B.; Mattsson, B. Two sides of the coin—General Practitioners' experience of working in multidisciplinary teams. *J. Interpret. Care* **2008**, *22*, 5–16. [CrossRef]

45. Johnson, P.; Wistow, G.; Schulz, R.; Hardy, B. Interagency and interprofessional collaboration in community care: The interdependence of structures and values. *J. Interpret. Care* **2003**, *17*, 69–83.

46. Department of Health. *Equity and Excellence: Liberating the NHS*; Department of Health: London, UK, 2010.

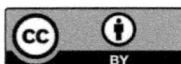

nutrients

MDPI

Article

Serum Phosphorus Levels in Premature Infants Receiving a Donor Human Milk Derived Fortifier

Katherine E. Chetta *, Amy B. Hair, Keli M. Hawthorne and Steven A. Abrams

USDA/ARS Children's Nutrition Research Center, Department of Pediatrics, Section of Neonatology, Baylor College of Medicine, Texas Children's Hospital, Houston, TX 77030, USA; abhair@bcm.edu (A.B.H.); kelih@bcm.edu (K.M.H.); sabrams@bcm.edu (S.A.B.)

* Author to whom correspondence should be addressed; kewiley@bcm.edu; Tel.: +1-832-826-3719.

Received: 13 November 2014; Accepted: 30 March 2015; Published: 9 April 2015

Abstract: An elevated serum phosphorus (P) has been anecdotally described in premature infants receiving human milk fortified with donor human milk-derived fortifier (HMDF). No studies have prospectively investigated serum P in premature infants receiving this fortification strategy. In this single center prospective observational cohort study, extremely premature infants $\leq$1250 grams (g) birth weight (BW) were fed an exclusive human milk-based diet receiving HMDF and serum P levels were obtained. We evaluated 93 infants with a mean gestational age of 27.5 $\pm$ 2.0 weeks (Mean $\pm$ SD) and BW of 904 $\pm$ 178 g. Seventeen infants (18.3%) had at least one high serum P level with a mean serum P of 9.2 $\pm$ 1.1 mg/dL occurring at 19 $\pm$ 11 days of life. For all infants, the highest serum P was inversely correlated to the day of life of the infant ($p < 0.001$, $R^2 = 0.175$) and positively correlated with energy density of HMDF ($p = 0.035$). Serum P was not significantly related to gender, BW, gestational age, or days to full feeds. We conclude that the incidence of hyperphosphatemia was mild and transient in this population. The risk decreased with infant age and was unrelated to gender, BW, or ethnicity.

Keywords: neonate; phosphorus; hyperphosphatemia; human milk; exclusive human milk-based diet; human milk-derived fortifier; prematurity; creatinine; donor milk; very low birth weight

1. Introduction

Human milk is the optimal source of nutrition for all infants, including preterm ones. The American Academy of Pediatrics (AAP) recommends that all infants <1500 g birth weight (BW) should receive human milk appropriately fortified [1]. An exclusive human-milk based diet is defined as mother's own milk (or pasteurized donor milk when mother's own milk is unavailable) fortified with a donor human milk-derived fortifier (HMDF), containing no preterm formula or cow milk protein-based fortifiers. This approach provides advantages over cow milk-containing products providing optimal growth rates, a lower rate of necrotizing enterocolitis, and decreased days of parenteral nutrition. Additionally, such an approach leads to lowered sepsis rates, decreased mortality, and shorter hospital stays [2–7].

Extremely premature infants are susceptible to growth failure, metabolic growth abnormalities, and poor neurodevelopmental outcomes [5,8–11]. Common metabolic derangements of extremely premature infants including hypocalcemia, hyperphosphatemia, and hypomagnesemia are usually secondary to immature hormone responses and renal dysfunction [8]. There are no published reports investigating the sequential early postnatal mineral serum chemistries of very low birth weight infants receiving an exclusive human milk-based diet with HMDF. This study aimed to evaluate how an exclusive human milk-based diet with HMDF can affect the risk of electrolyte abnormalities, specifically serum phosphorus.

There have been anecdotal reports of hyperphosphatemia associated with HMDF in extremely low birth weight infants and some health care providers may be limiting their use of this product because of this concern. Because of the potential benefits of using an exclusive human milk-based diet, but concern about phosphorus metabolism, we chose to evaluate the incidence of hyperphosphatemia, hypophosphatemia and hypocalcemia in all infants <1250 g BW receiving this diet.

2. Experimental Section

Extremely premature infants were consecutively followed in this single-center prospective observational cohort study from August 2010 to December 2011. Inclusion criteria were: premature infants <37 weeks gestation, BW <1250 g, admitted within 48 h of birth, receiving an exclusive human milk-based diet, and achievement of full enteral feedings by 4 weeks of age. Infants were excluded who died within the first week of life and those who had major congenital anomalies. Infants were followed from birth until discharge and data were prospectively collected for growth and nutrition using pre-study defined variables and definitions [3].

As approved by the Institutional Review Board of Baylor College of Medicine and Affiliated Hospitals, consent was waived for this observational study. Our primary outcome of this study was to evaluate the metabolic derangements in phosphorus levels for infants receiving an exclusive human milk-based diet with HMDF. Specifically, study outcomes included the number of phosphorus levels, mean phosphorus level drawn per infant, mean peak phosphorus level, percentage of infants with hyperphosphatemia (serum phosphorus > 8.0 mg/dL), percentage of infants with hypophosphatemia (serum phosphorus < 4.8 mg/dL), the incidence of hyperphosphatemia in relationship to serum creatinine, the incidence of hypocalcemia during hyperphosphatemia, and the day of life of peak phosphorus levels.

2.1. Standardized Feeding Protocol

Infants received a standardized feeding protocol which has been previously published by our group [3]. Human milk was fortified with HMDF Prolact +4, Prolact +6, Prolact +8, or Prolact +10 (Prolacta Bioscience, Industry, CA, USA) with final energy concentrations of 24 kcal/oz, 26 kcal/oz, 28 kcal/oz, and 30 kcal/oz, respectively, based on expected human milk energy concentration of 20 kcal/oz. Each fortifier adds 64 mg/dL of phosphorus and 122 mg/dL of calcium. This is comparable to most cow milk protein-based human milk fortifiers with phosphorus contents ranging from 26 mg/dL to 67 mg/dL and calcium contents ranging from 38 mg/dL to 138 mg/dL [2,12].

2.2. Data Collection

Serum phosphorus levels were collected per unit protocol three days after stopping parenteral nutrition and repeated one week later if serum phosphorus was >8.0 mg/dL. Further serum phosphorus values were collected at the discretion of the attending clinician. The peak phosphorus level (or single highest phosphorus level for one infant) was recorded along with the corresponding the day of life, degree of calorie fortification (energy density), and the number of days after discontinuation of parenteral nutrition. All infants with serum phosphorus levels >8.0 mg/dL were assessed with a serum creatinine, serum calcium, and serum alkaline phosphatase level within three days if available. Normal and low serum phosphorus levels in all infants were collected with corresponding day of life. Serum phosphorus levels were treated as one value if separated by less than 2 days.

Only serum phosphorus levels drawn during the use of the HMDF were used in this study. Of infants with multiple serum phosphorus levels on record, the highest level was considered the peak serum phosphorus level. Of infants with only one serum phosphorus level on record, that level was used.

2.3. Statistical Analyses

Relationships among variables were evaluated using general linear modeling in which hyperphosphatemia was the primary outcome. Regression analysis was used to compare relationships between peak serum phosphorus and day of life, energy density of HMDF, and days to achieve full feeds. Additionally, comparisons between serum phosphorus and gender, BW, gestational age, race, and >750 g or below 750 g BW were completed with univariate regression analysis. Statistical significance was defined as $p < 0.05$. A *t*-test was performed to compare the serum phosphorus and serum creatinine between an infant group within five days of discontinuation of parenteral nutrition and a group five days after discontinuation of parenteral nutrition. Analyses were completed using SPSS 22.0 (SPSS Inc., Chicago, IL, USA). All data are mean ± standard deviation unless otherwise noted.

3. Results

Of 124 infants identified who initially met the inclusion criteria, 93 were included for the analysis. (Figure 1). The demographics and outcomes are shown in Tables 1 and 2. In total, 356 serum phosphorus values were drawn among the 93 infants. On average, serum phosphorus levels were drawn 3.8 times per infant. Sixteen infants had only one serum phosphorus level checked, while 29 infants had serum phosphorus levels drawn over four times during their course (Table 3). Of 356 discrete levels during the use of HMDF, 291 (81%) serum phosphorus levels were within normal limits. The mean peak serum phosphorus was 7.2 ± 1.3 mg/dL. One infant was excluded for extreme hyperphosphatemia (serum phosphorus 17.8 mg/dL) at 48 days of life and was considered an outlier secondary to developing an incarcerated hernia at that time. Two infants also had hypocalcemia at the time of a high serum phosphorus level.

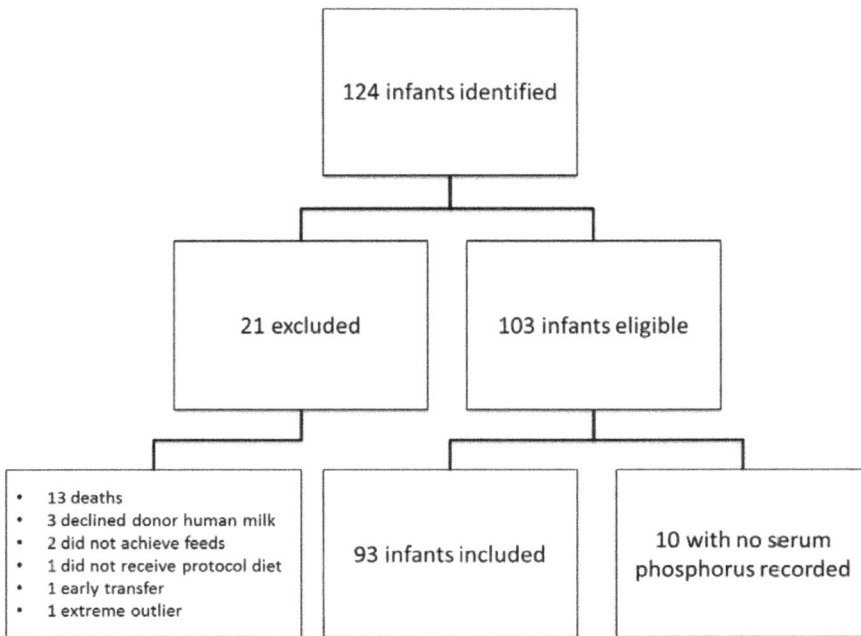

```
                    ┌──────────────────────────┐
                    │   124 infants identified │
                    └──────────────────────────┘
          ┌────────────────┐        ┌────────────────────────┐
          │  21 excluded   │        │  103 infants eligible  │
          └────────────────┘        └────────────────────────┘
┌─────────────────────────┐ ┌──────────────────────┐ ┌────────────────────┐
│ • 13 deaths             │ │                      │ │                    │
│ • 3 declined donor      │ │                      │ │  10 with no serum  │
│   human milk            │ │  93 infants included │ │ phosphorus recorded│
│ • 2 did not achieve feeds│ │                      │ │                    │
│ • 1 did not receive     │ │                      │ │                    │
│   protocol diet         │ │                      │ │                    │
│ • 1 early transfer      │ │                      │ │                    │
│ • 1 extreme outlier     │ │                      │ │                    │
└─────────────────────────┘ └──────────────────────┘ └────────────────────┘
```

Figure 1. Infants receiving the exclusive human milk-based diet were prospectively followed.

Table 1. Infant demographics and characteristics.

Demographics and Characteristics	Cohort n = 93
Birth weight, g	904 ± 178 *
Gestational age, weeks	27.5 ± 2.0
Male gender, n (%)	47 (51)
Race, % Black/White/Hispanic/Other	36, 25, 22, 10
Number of days to full 140 mL/kg/day feeds	16.0 ± 4.0
Inborn, n (%)	53 (57)
Antenatal steroids, n (%)	67 (72)

* Mean ± SD.

Table 2. Outcomes.

Outcomes	Cohort n = 93
Total serum phosphorus levels obtained	356
Mean number of serum phosphorus levels per infant	3.8 ± 2.5 *
Mean peak serum phosphorus level of all infants (mg/dL)	7.2 ± 1.3 *
Infants with high serum phosphorus (>8 mg/dL), n (%)	17 (18.3)
Total high serum phosphorus levels, n (%)	23 (7)
Infants with multiple high serum phosphorus levels, n (%)	5 (5)
Average high serum phosphorus level (mg/dL)	9.2 ± 1.1 *
Infants with low serum phosphorus (<4.8 mg/dL), n (%)	19 (20)
Total low serum phosphorus values (<4.8 mg/dL), n (%)	42 (13)
Infants with no serum phosphorus abnormalities, n (%)	64 (69)
Hypocalcemia occurring with high serum phosphorus level (serum calcium < 7.0 mg/dL or ionized calcium < 1.0 mmol/L), n	2

* Mean ± SD.

Table 3. Number of serum phosphorus levels recorded while on human milk-derived fortifier.

Number of Serum Phosphorus Levels Recorded Per Infant	n = 356
Only 1 level	16
2–3 levels	36
>4 levels	29
>6 levels	11

In the cohort, 17 infants (18.3%) had at least one laboratory result indicating hyperphosphatemia. Of these, five (5%) infants had more than one high level. Additionally, 19 (20%) infants had at least one episode of hypophosphatemia. Sixty-four (69%) of infants had all normal serum phosphorus levels. Of the infants with multiple high serum phosphorus levels, three infants had a serum creatinine over 1.0 mg/dL. Four of these infants received interventions (Table 4).

Ten (43%) of the high serum phosphorus levels were found to be within five days of transitioning off of parenteral nutrition. Eleven (45%) of the high serum phosphorus levels were associated with normal creatinine levels of <1 mg/dL, and of these 9 (81%) were within five days of the transition off of parenteral nutrition. Of the high serum phosphorus levels found five or more days after the transition off parenteral nutrition (12, 52%), half were associated with creatinine levels >1 mg/dL (Figure 2). Of the six high serum phosphorus levels associated with an elevated serum creatinine, the mean number of days from the transition off parenteral nutrition was 10.5 ± 5.0 days (Table 5). This is significantly different than the 11 high serum phosphorus levels associated with a normal creatinine found to be 4.9 ± 4.2 days from discontinuation of parenteral nutrition, p = 0.026.

Table 4. Outcomes of infants with multiple high serum phosphorus levels.

Infant	Serum Phosphorus	Intervention	Outcome	Serum Creatinine within 3 Days	Calorie Fortification (kcal/oz)
1	2 high values on day of life (DOL) 18 and 24 (both 8.2 mg/dL)	None	Serum phosphorus normalized on DOL 31	None	DOL 18: +4 DOL 24: +8
2	3 high values on DOL 13, 14, 19 (9.6, 8.1, and 9.3 mg/dL)	Treated for sepsis, found to have *Klebsiella* bacteremia	Serum phosphorus normalized on DOL 34	High creatinine 1.1 and 2.2 mg/dL, lowered DOL 24 (0.89 mg/dL)	DOL 13: +6 DOL 14: +8 DOL 19: +10
3	2 high values on DOL 12, 19 (8.4 and 10 mg/dL)	Worked up for sepsis. Cultures negative	Serum phosphorus normalized in subsequent checks on DOL 31, 52, 80	High creatinine 1.1 mg/dL lowered DOL 33 (0.55 mg/dL).	DOL 12: +6 DOL 19: +8 DOL 20: +10
4	2 high values on DOL 32, 45 (8.6 and 10.0 mg/dL)	Stopped HMDF for 1 day, worked up for sepsis	Serum phosphorus normalized in on DOL 50	High creatinine 1.3 mg/dL, normalized 0.4 mg/dL on DOL 114 (on formula)	DOL 32: +10 DOL 45: +10
5	2 high values on DOL 15, 23 (11.8 and 10.5 mg/dL)	HMDF held 1 day, DOL 16. Infant received IV calcium for hypocalcemia	Serum phosphorus normalized on DOL 20 and was normal on DOL 30 after resuming HDMF	Creatinine 0.74 and 0.91 mg/dL. Ionized calcium 0.84 mmol/L	DOL 15: +4 DOL 23: +10

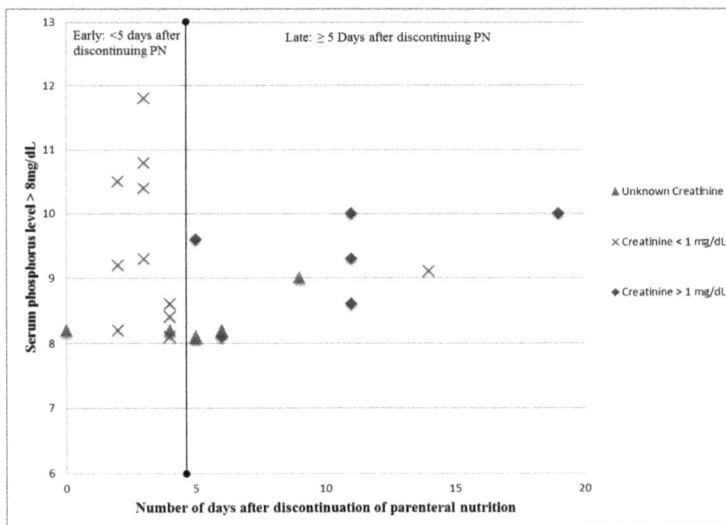

Figure 2. Comparison of creatinine levels in early *vs.* late hyperphosphatemia.

Table 5. Comparison of serum creatinine and high serum phosphorus levels.

Serum Creatinine (± 3 Days of High Serum Phosphorus Level)	Number of High Serum Phosphorus Levels ($n = 17$)	Mean Days after Parenteral Nutrition Discontinued
High (≥1 mg/dL)	6	10.5 ± 5.0 *
Normal (<1 mg/dL)	11	4.9 ± 4.2 *

* Significant difference between groups $p = 0.026$.

The serum phosphorus levels were closely associated with the age (day of life) of the infant ($p < 0.001$, $R^2 = 0.1746$) (Figure 3a,b). The serum phosphorus levels were also significantly correlated to energy density concentration of HMDF used ($p = 0.035$). The number of days the infant needed to achieve full feeds (140 mL/kg/day) and any intrinsic characteristics of the infant including gender,

BW, gestational age, race, or $\geq$750 g or < 750 g BW were not significantly associated with the risk of hyperphosphatemia.

Of 23 high serum phosphorus levels, 12 (52%) had serum calcium values drawn within three days. Ten of 12 levels were within normal limits. Two infants had laboratory evidence of hypocalcemia defined as < 7.0 mg/dL. One infant had a serum calcium level of 5.4 mg/dL and required a calcium infusion with the calcium level subsequently normalizing the next day. This infant had a creatinine level of 0.91 mg/dL and multiple high serum phosphorus levels. The other infant had a serum calcium level of 6.6 mg/dL which resolved three days later without supplementation. Alkaline phosphatase activity within 3 days was also recorded in 14 of the infants with high serum phosphorus levels and was found mildly elevated at 495 $\pm$ 215 mg/dL.

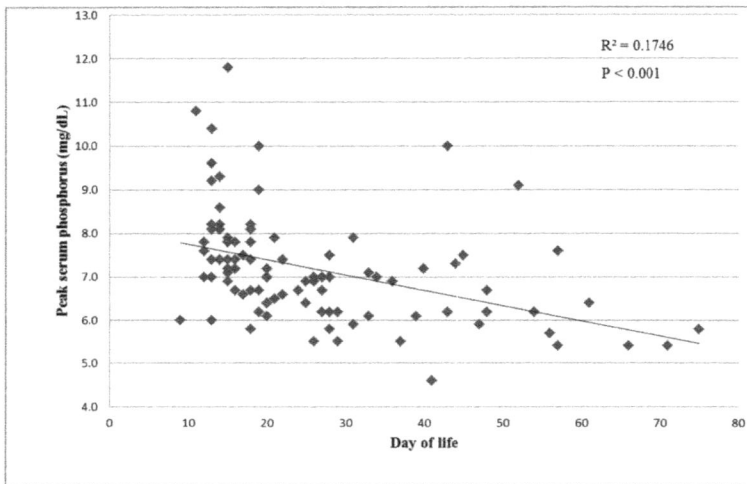

(a)

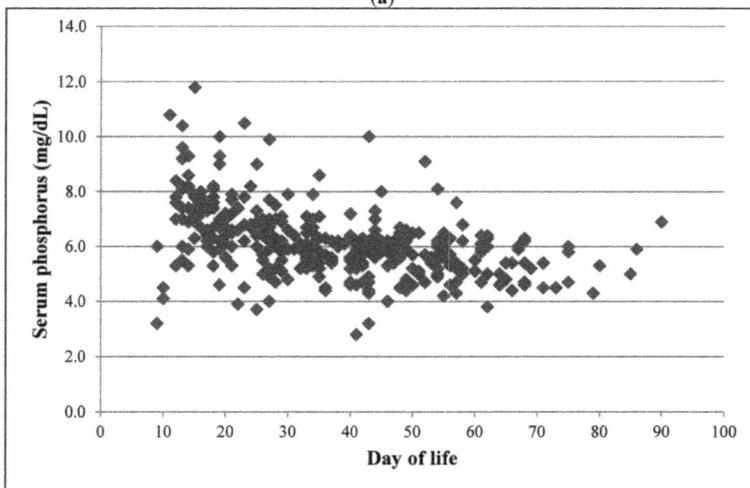

(b)

Figure 3. (a) Peak phosphorus level declines with day of life; (b) All serum phosphorus levels in 93 infants.

Very limited interventions were used in the infants with high serum phosphorus. The infants with multiple high serum phosphorus levels were more likely to receive interventions (Table 4) and often associated with high energy fortification (+8 and +10 kcal/oz). In four of the 17 infants with hyperphosphatemia, a decrease in daily feeding volume was made or the HMDF was stopped briefly (<3 days). These interventions coincided with a patent ductus arteriosus ligation and a clinically identified ileus associated with proven bloodstream infection for two infants. Most infants did not receive interventions, and all evidence of hyperphosphatemia resolved.

4. Discussion

Among 93 infants receiving an exclusive human milk-based diet, all serum phosphorus levels were analyzed with a focus on hyperphosphatemia. The average peak serum phosphorus level of infants receiving HMDF was <8.0 mg/dL. All infants received rapid advancement of feedings and increasingly high enteral phosphate loads.

Infants are susceptible to hypocalcemia and hypophosphatemia during prolonged parenteral nutrition and are often weaned to oral feedings rapidly as treatment [12]. Preterm infants fed unfortified mother's milk early in life develop hypophosphatemia and elevated alkaline phosphatase levels leading to rickets [12–16]. Supplementation may protect against hypophosphatemia as premature infants have a limited body pool of phosphorus from their soft tissues risking demineralization leading to fractures [12]. Both hypophosphatemia and hyperphosphatemia occurred at similar rates in this study.

Seventeen (18%) infants in this study had hyperphosphatemia. The hyperphosphatemia was mild and transient occurring mostly early in life after the discontinuation of parenteral nutrition with few exceptions. In 17 infants with high serum phosphorus levels, 13 (76%) did not require intervention. The four interventions were minor dietary changes (slowing, stopping feeds or HMDF) for a short period of time. Two infants also had a patent ductus arteriosus ligation and clinically identified ileus at the time of intervention.

Hyperphosphatemia largely occurred within five days from the discontinuation of parenteral nutrition, at approximately 10–15 days of life. The risk of hyperphosphatemia decreased as the infant aged. Several mechanisms could contribute to early peak serum phosphorus levels including increasing feeding volumes, high absorption (bioavailability) of the phosphorus loads and suppression of parathyroid function by calcium in parenteral nutrition [12]. Parathyroid hormone surges are smaller in very low birth weight infants but function improves with postnatal age as nephrogenesis continues through 34 weeks post-gestational age [8,17].

Hyperphosphatemia occurring more than five days after the discontinuation of parenteral nutrition (late) was often associated with serum creatinine ≥1 mg/dL, possibly signifying renal dysfunction and an inability to excrete ingested phosphorus [17,18]. Our study also found that the higher energy density of HMDF was significantly associated with hyperphosphatemia ($p = 0.025$). Feeds were highly fortified (+8 kcal/oz or +10 kcal/oz) after evidencing poor weight gain on full (140–150 mL/kg/day) feeds. Poor weight gain is an independent marker of underlying renal dysfunction [18]. Renal function should be investigated in infants with late hyperphosphatemia. Multiple high serum phosphorus levels were also a risk factor for intervention. One infant received a calcium infusion secondary to hypocalcemia during an episode of hyperphosphatemia. Alkaline phosphatase activity was mildly high on average, however it is a not a highly specific marker for bone mineral defects in premature infants [12].

A limitation of this observational study was the non-randomized nature of this cohort. The prospective nature of this study was its strength, investigating a large cohort of premature infants that were only using an exclusive human milk-based diet, while analyzing serum phosphorus as an outcome.

Nutrients **2015**, *7*, 2562–2573

5. Conclusions

An exclusive human milk-based diet provides phosphorus, supporting bone growth safely. Hyperphosphatemia was seen early in life with interventions being minor. Hypophosphatemia occurred with a similar frequency in this cohort. The risk of high serum phosphorus decreased with infant age unrelated to gender, BW, or ethnicity. An interesting point of this study was the correlation of high creatinine and late hyperphosphatemia. A clinician should be sensitive to serum phosphorus as a herald to renal dysfunction in these infants. When interpreting these interventions, recall that infants had comorbid renal dysfunction, sepsis, impending surgeries or a patent ductus arteriosus and had enteral feeds discontinued for those reasons rather than to treat hyperphosphatemia. Special consideration should be paid to electrolyte abnormalities when infants transition off of parenteral nutrition or demonstrate multiple high serum phosphorus levels as underlying renal dysfunction or rarely hypocalcemia may also be present. Monitoring serum phosphorus to assure a normalizing trend for this subset of premature infants receiving HMDF is supported.

Acknowledgments: We would like to thank Pam Gordon RNC-NIC and Geneva Shores RNC-LRN for their dedication to the project. Funding source: This project has been funded in part with federal funds from the USDA/ARS under Cooperative Agreement 58-6250-6-001 and National Center for Research Resources General Clinical Research for Children Grant RR00188. This work is a publication of the Department of Pediatrics, Baylor College of Medicine, and Texas Children's Hospital (Houston, TX, USA).

Author Contributions: Katherine E. Chetta designed the study, extracted the data, ran the statistics, authored and edited the paper. Amy B. Hair gained the IRB approval, mentored the design, edited the paper, extracted and verified the data extraction. Keli M. Hawthorne extracted the data and edited the paper. Steven A. Abrams mentored the design and edited the paper.

Conflicts of Interest: Katherine E. Chetta has no conflicts of interest. Amy B. Hair receives research support from Prolacta Bioscience for the Human Milk Cream Follow-up Study. She receives speaker honoraria from Prolacta Bioscience and Mead Johnson Nutrition. Keli M. Hawthorne receives speaker honoraria from Mead Johnson Nutrition and Abbott Nutrition. Steven A. Abrams receives research support from Mead Johnson Nutrition.

References

1. Section on Breastfeeding. Breastfeeding and the use of human milk. *Pediatrics* **2012**, *115*, 496. [CrossRef]
2. Sullivan, S.; Schanler, R.J.; Kim, J.H.; Patel, A.L.; Trawoger, R.; Kiechl-Kohlendorfer, U.; Chan, G.M.; Blanco, C.L.; Abrams, S.; Cotten, C.M.; *et al.* An exclusively human milk-based diet is associated with a lower rate of necrotizing enterocolitis than a diet of human milk and bovine milk-based products. *J. Pediatr.* **2010**, *156*, 562–567.e1.
3. Hair, A.B.; Hawthorne, K.M.; Chetta, K.E.; Abrams, S.A. Human milk feeding supports adequate growth in infants ≤1250 grams birth weight. *BMC Res. Notes* **2013**, *6*, 459. [CrossRef]
4. Ganapathy, V.; Hay, J.W.; Kim, J.H. Costs of necrotizing enterocolitis and cost-effectiveness of exclusively human milk-based products in feeding extremely premature infants. *Breastfeed. Med.* **2012**, *7*, 29–37. [CrossRef] [PubMed]
5. Abrams, S.A.; Schanler, R.J.; Lee, M.L.; Rechtman, D.J. Greater mortality and morbidity in extremely preterm infants fed a diet containing cow milk protein products. *Breastfeed. Med.* **2014**, *9*, 281–285. [CrossRef] [PubMed]
6. De Silva, A.; Jones, P.; Spencer, S. Does human milk reduce infection rates in preterm infants? A systematic review. *Arch. Dis. Child. Fetal and Neonatal Ed.* **2004**, *89*, F509–F513. [CrossRef]
7. Cristofalo, E.A.; Schanler, R.J.; Blanco, C.L.; Sullivan, S.; Trawoeger, R.; Kiechl-Kohlendorfer, U.; Dudell, G.; Rechtman, D.J.; Lee, M.L.; Lucas, A.; *et al.* Randomized trial of exclusive human milk *versus* preterm formula diets in extremely premature infants. *J. Pediatr.* **2013**, *163*, 1592–1595.e1.
8. Buonocore, G.; Bracci, R.; Weindling, M. *Neonatology: A Practical Approach to Neonatal Diseases*; Springer: Verlag, Italy, 2011.
9. Meinzen-Derr, J.; Poindexter, B.; Wrage, L.; Morrow, A.; Stoll, B.; Donovan, E. Role of human milk in extremely low birth weight infants' risk of necrotizing enterocolitis or death. *J. Perinatol.* **2008**, *29*, 57–62. [CrossRef] [PubMed]

10. Vohr, B.R.; Poindexter, B.B.; Dusick, A.M.; McKinley, L.T.; Wright, L.L.; Langer J.C.; Poole, W.K. Beneficial effects of breast milk in the neonatal intensive care unit on the developmental outcome of extremely low birth weight infants at 18 months of age. *Pediatrics* **2006**, *118*, e115–e123. [CrossRef] [PubMed]

11. Hawthorne, K.; Griffin, I.; Abrams, S. Current issues in nutritional management of very low birth weight infants. *Miner. Pediatr.* **2004**, *56*, 359–372.

12. Tsang, R.C.; Uauy, R.; Koletzko, B.; Zlotkin, S. *Nutrition of the Preterm Infant: Scientific Basis and Practical Guidelines*; Digital Educational Publishing: Cincinnati, OH, USA, 2005.

13. Schanler, R.J. The use of human milk for premature infants. *Pediatr. Clin. North. Am* **2001**, *48*, 207–219. [CrossRef] [PubMed]

14. Rowe, J.; Rowe, D.; Horak, E.; Spackman, T.; Saltzman, R.; Robinson, S.; Philipps, A.; Raye, J. Hypophosphatemia and hypercalciuria in small premature infants fed human milk: Evidence for inadequate dietary phosphorus. *J. Pediatr.* **1984**, *104*, 112–117. [CrossRef] [PubMed]

15. Atkinson, S.A.; Radde, I.C.; Anderson, G.H. Macromineral balances in premature infants fed their own mothers' milk or formula. *J. Pediatr.* **1983**, *102*, 99–106. [CrossRef] [PubMed]

16. Schanler, R.; Rifka, M. Calcium, phosphorus and magnesium needs for the low-birth-weight infant. *Acta Paediatr.* **1994**, *83*, 111–116. [CrossRef]

17. Andreoli, S.P. Acute renal failure in the newborn. *Semin. Perinatol.* **2004**, *28*, 112–123. [CrossRef] [PubMed]

18. Haycock, G.B. Management of acute and chronic renal Failure in the newborn. *Semin. Neonatol.* **2003**, *8*, 325–334. [CrossRef] [PubMed]

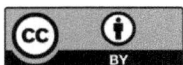

nutrients

[MDPI]

Review

Enteral Nutrition in Pancreaticoduodenectomy: A Literature Review

Salvatore Buscemi [1,2,†,*], **Giuseppe Damiano** [3], **Vincenzo D. Palumbo** [2,3,4], **Gabriele Spinelli** [2], **Silvia Ficarella** [2], **Giulia Lo Monte** [5], **Antonio Marrazzo** [2] and **Attilio I. Lo Monte** [2,3,†]

[1] School of Oncology and Experimental Surgery, University of Palermo, via Del Vespro 129, 90127 Palermo, Italy

[2] Department of Surgical, Oncological and Dentistry Studies, University of Palermo, via Del Vespro 129, 90127 Palermo, Italy; vincenzopalumbo84@libero.it (V.D.P.); gabriele.spinelli@unipa.it (G.S.); silvia.ficarella@gmail.com (S.F.); antonio.marrazzo@unipa.it (A.M.); attilioignazio.lomonte@unipa.it (A.I.L.M.)

[3] "P.Giaccone", University Hospital, School of Medicine, School of Biotechnology, University of Palermo, via Del Vespro 129, 90127 Palermo, Italy; giuse.damiano@gmail.com

[4] School of Surgical Biotechnology and Regenerative Medicine in Organ Failure, University of Palermo, via Del Vespro 129, 90127 Palermo, Italy

[5] School of Biotechnology, University of Palermo, via Del Vespro 129, 90127 Palermo, Italy; giulialom@virgilio.it

* Author to whom correspondence should be addressed; buscemi.salvatore@gmail.com; Tel.: +39 3357593376.

† These authors contributed equally to this work.

Received: 30 November 2014; Accepted: 15 April 2015; Published: 30 April 2015

Abstract: Pancreaticoduodenectomy (PD) is considered the gold standard treatment for periampullory carcinomas. This procedure presents 30%–40% of morbidity. Patients who have undergone pancreaticoduodenectomy often present perioperative malnutrition that is worse in the early postoperative days, affects the process of healing, the intestinal barrier function and the number of postoperative complications. Few studies focus on the relation between enteral nutrition (EN) and postoperative complications. Our aim was to perform a review, including only randomized controlled trial meta-analyses or well-designed studies, of evidence regarding the correlation between EN and main complications and outcomes after pancreaticoduodenectomy, as delayed gastric emptying (DGE), postoperative pancreatic fistula (POPF), postpancreatectomy hemorrhage (PPH), length of stay and infectious complications. Several studies, especially randomized controlled trial have shown that EN does not increase the rate of DGE. EN appeared safe and tolerated for patients after PD, even if it did not reveal any advantages in terms of POPF, PPH, length of stay and infectious complications.

Keywords: Enteral nutrition; pancreaticoduodenectomy; delayed gastric emptying; postoperative pancreatic fistula; postpancreatectomy hemorrhage

---

1. Introduction

Gastrointestinal surgery involving intestinal resection and anastomosis often requires a period of starvation or "nil by mouth", while new anastomosis heal. The aim of this strategy is to allow time for intestinal motility to return to normal, and to protect anastomosis from the stress of introducing oral fluids and diet [1]. Hepatobiliary surgery is usually performed in malnourished patients, and this condition if severe can be associated with a higher incidence of complications [2,3]. Pancreaticoduodenectomy (PD) is considered the gold standard treatment for periampullary carcinomas. This procedure is one of the most invasive operations in abdominal surgery and postoperative morbidity ranges between 30% and 40% [4]. PD results in a loss of gastric pacemaker and a partial pancreatic resection, and leads to a high incidence of postoperative malnutrition. The surgical trauma increases immune system suppression. The surgical injury as well as the malnutrition can provide bad postoperative outcomes. The malnutrition is worse in the early postoperative days, affects the process of healing, the intestinal barrier function and the incidence of postoperative complications [5,6]. Perioperative nutrition supplements, including enteral nutrition (EN) and total parental nutrition (TPN), have demonstrated to be effective in improving clinical outcomes and in decreasing the incidence of postoperative complications in major abdominal surgery [7,8], repairing immune function and reducing risk of sepsis, especially early EN [9,10].

Postoperative nutritional support can improve clinical outcome in patients underwent PD resolving the malnutrition status of the patients. Early EN after PD can influence both the endocrine and the exocrine function of the gland and can stimulate the pancreatic and bile secretion [11].

On the other hand, several studies reported different results and this is clear by reading the current nutritional guidelines. The current guidelines of the European Society for Parenteral and Enteral Nutrition recommend routine use of early enteral nutrition in patients undergoing major gastrointestinal surgery for cancer, including PD [12]. In contrast, the current American Society for Parenteral and Enteral Nutrition guidelines recommend postoperative nutritional support only in patients who are unlikely to meet their nutrient needs orally for a period of 7–10 days, which is not necessarily the case after PD [13]. Both of these guidelines are based on a few studies concerning pancreatic cancer.

The aim of this review is to focus on specific evidence regarding the enteral feeding strategy and the correlation between EN, main complications and outcomes after PD.

2. Enteral Nutrition and Outcomes after Pancreaticoduodenectomy

In 2006, Goonetilleke and Siriwardena published a systematic review regarding perioperative nutritional support after PD. The Authors examined 10 studies, investigating nutritional support after PD, and concluded favorably about EN, also showing that early mandatory, postoperative TPN was not associated with improved outcomes. The review of the Authors also implied that administration of postoperative EN helps to decrease infectious complications [14].

Further studies have been published after 2006, focusing on the relation between EN and postoperative complications, like delayed gastric emptying (DGE), postoperative pancreatic fistula (POPF), postpancreatectomy hemorrhage (PPH), infectious complications or clinical outcome, such as length of hospitalization.

2.1. Delayed Gastric Emptying (DGE)

Gastroparesis is one of the most important complications after PD, with a reported incidence between 19% and 44% even in centers dedicated to pancreatic surgery [15,16].

According to the International Study Group of Pancreas Surgery (ISGPS), delayed gastric emptying (DGE) is defined as the need of a nasogastric tube (NGT) for >3 days or the need of reinsert the NGT for persistent vomiting after surgery [17]. The ISGPS also classifies the severity of DGE as grade A: NGT required for 4–7 days or reinsertion after postoperative day (POD) 3 or inability to tolerate solid oral intake by POD 7; grade B: NGT required for 8–14 days or inability to tolerate solid oral intake by POD 14; grade C: NGT required for >14 days or inability to tolerate solid food by POD 21 [17].

The pathophysiological mechanism contributing to the development of gastroparesis is unknown. The mechanism is probably multifactorial. Likely factors involved in DGE after PD may be the presence of pancreatic fibrosis [18], intraperitoneal inflammation secondary to postoperative complications [19,20], gastrointestinal reconstruction [21,22], removal of the duodenum [23] or extended lymph node dissection [24,25]. Several authors suggest that DGE is also caused by gastric denervation due to the loss of parasympathetic nerves, resulting in the reduction of peristalsis and secretion of motilin [26]. Ligation of the right gastric and gastroduodenal arteries could be responsible for pylorus and antrum ischemia contributing to postoperative pylorospasm in pylorus-preserving

PD [27]. When gastroparesis occurs it is very difficult to anticipate the need for nutritional support, but feeding can be administrated directly to the jejunum [28].

Some studies reported no increase or even decrease in the incidence of gastroparesis after PD with early EN [29]. Tien *et al.* performed a prospective randomized trial to test the effectiveness of biliopancraetic diversion with modified Roux-en-Y gastrojejunostomy reconstruction and of EN to minimize impacts of DGE after PD. In total 257 patients with periampullay tumors were randomized and underwent PD. DGE occurred in 20 patients (16.3%) in the EN group and 27 patients (21.7%) in the control group. Although statistical analysis revealed no difference ($p = 0.27$) in DGE between groups, ISGPS grades of gastric stasis were significantly lower in the modified group than in the control group ($p = 0.001$) [30].

In another randomized controlled trial, Mack *et al.* reported the benefit of gastric decompression and enteral feeding through a double-lumen gastrojejunostomy tube. Prolonged gastroparesis occurred in 4 controls (25%) and in none of the patients who had gastrojejunostomy ($p = 0.03$). In the author's experience, the insertion of this kind of tube was found to be safe and feasible [31]. Although operative time was longer, no major problems occurred during tube insertion. Anyway, it is not clear if this result was due to the tube itself or to the efficacy of enteral nutrition.

In 2008 Grizas, comparing in a randomized controlled trial the effectiveness of the early enteral and natural nutrition after PD, did not notice any statistically significant difference in clinical or radiological manifestation of DGE between the two groups [32].

A recent meta-analysis of randomized controlled trial has been conducted to evaluate the safety and effectiveness of early enteral nutrition for patients after PD. Only four studies published in 2000 or later have been included in the analysis, involving 246 patients who underwent EN and 238 patients who underwent other nutritional routes. The rate of DGE in EN and other nutritional routes groups after PD was 15.9% and 18.9% respectively. Meta-analysis showed no statistically significant difference in DGE between EN and other nutritional routes group (OR, 0.89; 95% CI, 0.36–2.18; $p = 0.79$) [11]. Therefore, early EN would be tolerable for patients after PD, without increased gastroparesis. These results are in line with the previous studies regarding the effect of EN to DGE. However, this meta-analysis presents some limitations, due to the lack of relevant information in the original works. First of all, the definition of gastroparesis in the included studies was not always in according to DGE definition of ISGPS; the kind of tube placed in the jejunum and used for EN differed in the studies; the type of EN, cyclical or continuous, is important and it was not specified; van Berge Henegouwen *et al.* performed a randomized trial showing that in patients undergoing pylorus-preserving PD, the use of cyclical infusion of EN (stopped for 6 h overnight) had some advantages over continuous (24 h) EN [33]. Finally, the content of nutritional supplementation significantly influences the outcome. Gianotti *et al.*, performing randomized trial, reported that an enteral formula enriched with arginine, omega-3 fatty acids and RNA statistically reduced postoperative complications and length of hospitalization compared to standard enteral nutrition or TPN [34]. In addition, one of the studies in the meta-analysis did not report the nutritional route of the control group [31].

As reported, DGE is a multifactorial complication and still remains unclear which factors are related to gastroparesis. DGE incidence has been shown to be closely associated with postoperative pancreatic fistula, hemorrhage and abdominal collection [19]. In the study of Rayar *et al.*, protective factors reducing DGE were reported to be EN ($p = 0.047$, OR = 0.56) as well as the patient's age ($p < 0.01$, OR = 1.01) and acute pancreatitis history prior to PD ($p = 0.013$, OR = 0.32) [35]. According to the authors, potential mechanisms of EN may be the mechanical effects of the nasojejunal tube across the anastomosis, which can stimulate the motility of the stomach and jejunum, or the stimulation of bowel peristalsis by the input of nutritional liquids [35,36].

It is clear therefore that even if some authors reported in previous study that EN was associated with a higher frequency of DGE [37], recent studies, especially randomized controlled trials, have shown that EN does not increase the rate of DGE [30–32,34]. Further studies and well-designed trials need to be conducted to demonstrate if EN is superior to early oral intake in preventing DGE after PD.

2.2. Postoperative Pancreatic Fistula

Postoperative pancreatic fistula (POPF) is another common complication in PD patients, with rates up to 12% in specialized centers [38].

According to ISGPS definition, POPF is defined as output via an operatively placed drain (or a subsequently placed percutaneous drain) of any measurable volume of drain fluid on or after postoperative day 3, with an amylase content greater than three times the upper serum value [39]. Okabayashi *et al.* investigating 100 patients who underwent PD from 1999 to 2007, identified, as independent parameter correlating with occurrence of POPF, not having early EN through the jejunostomy catheter (*p* = 0.007) [40]. In the series, this finding indicates that early EN was associated with a reduced incidence of fistula. The same Author, in a previous study, compared the outcome of patients underwent PD and were then either managed with early EN (starting on the day after surgery) or late EN (starting 7–14 days after surgery). In that study, early EN was associated not only with a decreased incidence of POPF, but also with sustained serum concentration of total protein and albumin, maintenance of body mass index, early restoration of peripheral lymphocyte count, and a shorter period of hospitalization [29].

In his retrospective study, Rayar did not detect any difference in the incidence of POPF between patients received EN until total oral alimentation compared to patients who did not receive EN and were orally fed after removing the nasogastric tube [35]. However, the incidence of POPF in control group may have been underestimated because routine amylase dosage in abdominal drain has only been performed since 2005.

Liu *et al.* observed a low rate of POPF in EN group compared to TPN group (*p* = 0.039). The reason of this difference remains unclear and requires further studies, hopefully with a major number of patients [41].

No difference in POPF rate has been reported in trials conducted comparing EN with other nutritional routes [30–32,42,43], even if only two studies reported the use of ISGPS definition of POPF [30,42]. Also, the meta-analysis of Shen, including POPF in intra-abdominal complication, showed no significant difference in intra-abdominal complications between EN and other nutritional routes [11]. However, in these studies EN appeared safe and tolerated for the patients after PD, even if it did not reveal any advantages in terms of POPF rate.

2.3. Postpancreatectomy Hemorrhage

Postpancreatectomy hemorrhage (PPH) is one of the most important complications after PD, with a reported incidence between 1% and 8% even in centers specializing in pancreatic surgery [44].

In 2007, the International Study Group of Pancreatic Surgery (ISGPS) proposed a new classification system of PPH with the aims to allow a proper diagnosis and to evaluate the severity of the hemorrhage; three different grades of PPH (grades A, B, and C) were defined according to the time of onset, site of bleeding, severity, and clinical impact [44]. As well known, PPH is also significantly related to many risk factors, such as POPF [45].

The retrospective study of Rayar reports a statistically significant difference in the incidence of PPH between the EN group and the control group (8% *vs.* 20%, respectively, *p* = 0.008). No significant differences were reported regarding grade and localization of the hemorrhage [35].

Concerning the protective factors for PPH, in 2011 Liu, comparing in randomized controlled trial the effectiveness of early enteral *vs.* total parental nutrition after PD, noticed that the incidence of PPH was significantly reduced in the EN group (1 case *vs.* 9 cases, respectively, *p* = 0.021) [41]. However the study was based on a small cohort (60 patients), and the inclusion criteria was so strict that most patients were in relatively good health conditions.

The meta-analysis of Shen reported only the rate of intra-abdominal complications, including also the PPH. Meta-analysis showed no statistically significant difference in intra-abdominal complications between EN and other nutritional routes (OR, 0.82; 95% CI, 0.53–1.26; *p* = 0.37) [11]. Due to the lack of relevant information in the original works, a subgroup analysis on PPH was not be performed; moreover, only one study used ISGPS's definition to grade hemorrhage [30].

Regarding the influence of EN on the incidence of PPH, more studies are required, involving more patients and using the recommendations and the grades of ISGPS.

2.4. Length of Stay

One hundred and twenty-one patients with suspected operable upper gastrointestinal cancer (including 54 esophageal, 38 gastric and 29 pancreatic neoplasms) were randomized to receive early EN or control management (nil by mouth and IV fluids) in a prospective multicentre randomized controlled trial [43]. The results showed a clear advantage for EN in terms of length of stay (LOS) both intention-to-treat and per-protocol analysis (16 days *vs.* 19 days, $p = 0.023$ and $p = 0.011$, respectively) and there were no statistically significant differences between the two groups for hospital readmission after discharge. Even if it did not include only patients with pancreatic cancer, the importance of this study is that it represents the first adequately powered prospective randomized trial of early EN *vs.* "nil by mouth" in patients undergoing upper gastrointestinal resectional surgery in the United Kingdom.

Regarding the use of EN after PD to reduce the LOS, while several retrospective studies did not report any clear advantages compared to other nutritional route [35,46], Zhu *et al.* demonstrated a lower LOS combining EN with parental nutrition compared to TPN postoperative regimen (13.2 days *vs.* 16.8 days, $p < 0.05$) [47].

More evidence could be obtained from the meta-analysis of randomized controlled trial conducted by Shen [11]. Only two trials provided information regarding postoperative hospital stay, involving 388 patients [30,34]. EN was not associated with a significantly shorter LOS than other nutritional route ($p = 0.74$). As we have reported, this meta-analysis presents some limits, first of all, one of the two trials examined was published in 2000 [34], and several improvements have been obtained from 2000 to the present days regarding the postoperative management after PD. In addition, the trial of Tien included patients underwent biliopancreatic diversion with modified Roux-en-Y gastrojejunostomy reconstruction, so it is difficult to establish if the results are due to the modified surgical procedure or to the EN [30].

In a randomized controlled trial by Mack *et al.*, LOS was reduced by routine double-lumen gastrojejunostomy tube feeding compared to "standard care" (11.5 days *vs.* 15.8 days respectively, $p = 0.01$). However, it was not specified what the "standard care" meant, in fact patients in the control group were treated in according to the operating surgeon's routine, including insertion of nasogastric tube and administration of nutritional support if the surgeon felt it was indicated, and the route of administration was also dictated by the surgeon's routine practice [31]. It remains unclear how the results seen in the study were secondary to the tube itself or to the effects of EN. Furthermore, this study appeared to be underpowered (only 36 patients enrolled) to demonstrate improvements in outcomes typically studied in enteral feeding trial.

In the systematic review of Gerritsen *et al.*, including 15 studies of different feeding route after PD (7 randomized trials, 7 cohort studies and 1 case-control study), mean length of hospital stay was shorter in the oral diet and gastrojejunostomy tube groups, both at 15 days, followed by 19 days in jejunostomy tube, 20 days in the TPN and 25 days in the nasojejunal tube groups [48].

Several large studies found good results with a normal oral diet (without routine nutritional support) after PD. Yermilov *et al.* reviewed the California Cancer Registry (1194–2003) for outcomes of 1873 patients who underwent PD for adenocarcinoma receiving either parental feeding (14%), jejunostomy tube feeding (23%) or an oral diet without supplemental nutritional support (63%). They showed a significantly shorter LOS in the normal diet cohort [49].

A recent review suggested that implementation of a fast-track protocol, including early oral feeding, in pancreatic surgery could lead to reduce LOS and reduced costs without an increase in morbidity, mortality or readmission rates [50].

Future randomized studies should compare outcomes of a routine oral diet (with on demand nasojejunal feeding) with routine nasojejunal feeding after PD.

2.5. Infectious Complications

Several studies reported that the use of EN reduced the risk of infections. A meta-analysis by Braunschweig *et al.*, combining 27 randomized controlled trials (n = 1828), found a significantly lower risk of infections with enteral nutrition (RR = 0.64) compared to parental feeding. [51].

A systematic review and meta-analysis of randomized controlled trials comparing any type of enteral feeding started within 24 h after surgery with nil by mouth management in elective gastrointestinal surgery showed that early EN reduced the risk of any type of infection (relative risk 0.72, 95% confidence interval 0.54 to 0.98, p = 0.036) [52].

In the prospective randomized controlled trial by Barlow *et al.* of early EN *vs.* "nil by mouth" in patients undergoing upper gastrointestinal resectional surgery, operative morbidity was less common after early EN compared to control management (nil by mouth and IV fluids) (32.8% *vs.* 50.9 respectively, p = 0.044). In particular the study showed a significantly difference in the rate of wound and chest infections (p = 0.017 and p = 0.036, respectively) [43].

Even if these data suggest that the use of EN presents some advantages in terms of reduction of infectious complications, these studies did not include patients underwent only PD. Regarding the use of EN after PD, only two trials revealed advantages in terms of infectious complications [32,34]. Gianotti *et al.* performing randomized trial, reported that an enteral formula enriched with arginine, omega-3 fatty acids and RNA reduced statistically the infectious complications compared to TPN (8.4% *vs.* 22.1% respectively, p = 0.04) [34]. As well Grizas, comparing the effectiveness of the early enteral and natural nutrition regimen (from liquid to solid diet in the first five postoperative days) after PD, noticed a higher rate of postoperative complications in the natural nutrition group (53.3% *vs.* 23.3% respectively, p = 0.03) with an odds ratio of 3.8. This difference seems to occur due to higher incidence of infectious complications in the natural nutrition group (46.7% *vs.* 16.7% respectively, p = 0.025), with an odds ratio of 4.4 [32].

Hypothesis that EN is beneficial in reducing infectious complications is supported by the evidence that modifications in the mucosal defense have been implicated as important factors affecting infectious complications in critically ill patients [53]. EN influences the ability of gut-associated lymphoid tissue to maintain mucosal immunity. Both route and type of nutrition influence antibacterial respiratory tract immunity [54].

Despite these data, the recent meta-analysis of a randomized controlled trial by Shen *et al.* showed no significant difference in infections between early EN and other nutritional routes after PD [11].

Further and more powerful trials are probably required to understand the real benefit of EN in the reduction of infectious complications.

3. Conclusions

This review summarized the available evidence on early EN after PD, which appears to be safe and tolerated in patients but does not have clear advantages reducing DGE, POPF, PPH, infectious complications and LOS. Future large-scale, high-quality, multicenter trials are still required to clarify the role of early EN after PD.

Acknowledgments: The authors acknowledge the reviewers for their insightful comments and recommendations.

Author Contributions: All authors equally contributed to the preparation of the manuscript and have approved the final version.

Conflicts of Interest: The authors declare no conflict of interest.

References

1. Lewis, S.J.; Andersen, H.K.; Thomas, S. Early enteral nutrition within 24 h of intestinal surgery *vs.* later commencement of feeding: A systematic review and meta-analysis. *J. Gastrointest. Surg.* **2009**, *13*, 569–575. [CrossRef] [PubMed]
2. Nygren, J.; Thorell, A.; Ljungqvist, O. New developments facilitating nutritional intake after gastrointestinal surgery. *Curr. Opin. Clin. Nutr. Metab. Care* **2003**, *6*, 593–597. [CrossRef] [PubMed]
3. Braga, M.; Ljungqvist, O.; Soeters, P.; Fearon, K.; Weimann, A.; Bozzetti, F.; ESPEN. ESPEN Guidelines on Parenteral Nutrition: Surgery. *Clin. Nutr.* **2009**, *28*, 378–386. [CrossRef]
4. Wente, M.N.; Shrikhande, S.V.; Müller, M.W.; Diener, M.K.; Seiler, C.M.; Friess, H.; Büchler, M.W. Pancreaticojejunostomy *vs.* pancreaticogastrostomy: Systematic review and meta-analysis. *Am. J. Surg.* **2007**, *193*, 171–183. [CrossRef]
5. Correia, M.I.; Caiaffa, W.T.; da Silva, A.L.; Waitzberg, D.L. Risk factors for malnutrition in patients undergoing gastroenterological and hernia surgery: An analysis of 374 patients. *Nutr. Hosp.* **2001**, *16*, 59–64. [PubMed]
6. Schnelldorfer, T.; Adams, D.B. The effect of malnutrition on morbidity after Surgery for chronic pancreatitis. *Am. Surg.* **2005**, *71*, 466–472. [PubMed]
7. Braga, M.; Vignali, A.; Gianotti, L.; Cestari, A.; Profili, M.; Carlo, V.D. Immune and nutritional effects of early enteral nutrition after major abdominal operations. *Eur. J. Surg.* **1996**, *162*, 105–112. [PubMed]
8. Ziegler, T.R. Perioperative nutritional support in patients undergoing hepatectomy for hepatocellular carcinoma. *JPEN J. Parenter. Enter. Nutr.* **1996**, *20*, 91–92. [CrossRef]
9. Beier-Holgersen, R.; Boesby, S. Influence of postoperative enteral nutrition on postsurgical infections. *Gut* **1996**, *39*, 833–835. [CrossRef] [PubMed]
10. Slotwinski, R.; Olszewski, W.L.; Slotkowski, M.; Lech, G.; Zaleska, M.; Slotwinska, S.M.; Krasnodebski, W.I. Can the interleukin-1 receptor antagonist (IL-1ra) be a marker of anti-inflammatory response to enteral immunonutrition in malnourished patients after pancreaticoduodenectomy? *J. Pancreas.* **2007**, *8*, 759–769.
11. Shen, Y.; Jin, W. Early enteral nutrition after pancreatoduodenectomy: A meta-analysis of randomized controlled trials. *Langenbecks Arch. Surg.* **2013**, *398*, 817–823. [CrossRef] [PubMed]
12. Weimann, A.; Braga, M.; Harsanyi, L.; Laviano, A.; Ljungqvist, O.; Soeters, P.; German Society for Nutritional Medicine; Jauch, K.W.; Kemen, M.; Hiesmayr, J.M.; *et al.* ESPEN Guidelines on Enteral Nutrition: Surgery including organ transplantation. *Clin. Nutr.* **2006**, *25*, 224–244. [CrossRef]
13. ASPEN Board of Directors and the Clinical Guidelines Task Force. Guidelines for the use of parenteral and enteral nutrition in adult and pediatric patients. *J. Parenter. Enter. Nutr.* **2002**, *26*, 1SA–138SA.
14. Goonetilleke, K.S.; Siriwardena, A.K. Systematic review of perioperative nutritional supplementation in patients undergoing pancreaticoduodenectomy. *J. Pancreas.* **2006**, *7*, 5–13.
15. Qu, H.; Sun, G.R.; Zhou, S.Q.; He, Q.S. Clinical risk factors of delayed gastric emptying in patients after pancreaticoduodenectomy: a systematic review and meta-analysis. *Eur. J. Surg. Oncol.* **2013**, *39*, 213–223. [CrossRef] [PubMed]
16. Yeo, C.J.; Cameron, J.L.; Sohn, T.A.; Lillemoe, K.D.; Pitt, H.A.; Talamini, M.A.; Hruban, R.H.; Ord, S.E.; Sauter, P.K.; Coleman, J.; *et al.* Six hundred fifty consecutive pancreaticoduodenectomies in the 1990s: Pathology, complications, and outcomes. *Ann. Surg.* **1997**, *226*, 248–257. [CrossRef]
17. Wente, M.N.; Bassi, C.; Dervenis, C.; Fingerhut, A.; Gouma, D.J.; Izbicki, J.R.; Neoptolemos, J.P.; Padbury, R.T.; Sarr, M.G.; Traverso, L.W.; *et al.* Delayed gastric emptying (DGE) after pancreatic surgery: A suggested definition by the International Study Group of Pancreatic Surgery (ISGPS). *Surgery* **2007**, *142*, 761–768. [CrossRef]
18. Murakami, H.; Suzuki, H.; Nakamura, T. Pancreatic fibrosis correlates with delayed gastric emptying after pylorus-preserving pancreaticoduodenectomy with pancreaticogastrostomy. *Ann. Surg.* **2002**, *235*, 240–245. [CrossRef] [PubMed]
19. Riediger, H.; Makowiec, F.; Schareck, W.D.; Hopt, U.T.; Adam, U. Delayed gastric emptying after pylorus-preserving pancreatoduodenectomy is strongly related to other postoperative complications. *J. Gastrointest. Surg.* **2003**, *7*, 758–765. [CrossRef] [PubMed]
20. Park, Y.C.; Kim, S.W.; Jang, J.Y.; Ahn, Y.J.; Park, Y.H. Factors influencing delayed gastric emptying after pylorus-preserving pancreatoduodenectomy. *J. Am. Coll. Surg.* **2003**, *196*, 859–865. [CrossRef] [PubMed]

21. Goei, T.H.; van Berge Henegouwen, M.I.; Slooff, M.J.; van Gulik, T.M.; Gouma, D.J.; Eddes, E.H. Pylorus-preserving pancreatoduodenectomy: Influence of a Billroth I *vs.* a Billroth II type of reconstruction on gastric emptying. *Dig. Surg.* **2001**, *18*, 376–380. [CrossRef] [PubMed]

22. Takahata, S.; Ohtsuka, T.; Nabae, T.; Matsunaga, H.; Yokohata, K.; Yamaguchi, K.; Chijiiwa, K.; Tanaka, M. Comparison of recovery of gastric phase III motility and gastric juice output after different types of gastrointestinal reconstruction following pylorus-preserving pancreatoduodenectomy. *J. Gastroenterol.* **2002**, *37*, 596–603. [CrossRef] [PubMed]

23. Müller, M.W.; Friess, H.; Beger, H.G.; Kleeff, J.; Lauterburg, B.; Glasbrenner, B.; Riepl, R.L.; Büchler, M.W. Gastric emptying following pylorus-preserving whipple and duodenum-preserving pancreatic head resection in patients with chronic pancreatitis. *Am. J. Surg.* **1997**, *173*, 257–263. [CrossRef] [PubMed]

24. Yeo, C.J.; Cameron, J.L.; Sohn, T.A.; Coleman, J.; Sauter, P.K.; Hruban, R.H.; Pitt, H.A.; Lillemoe, K.D. Pancreaticoduodenectomy with or without extended retroperitoneal lymphadenectomy for periampullary adenocarcinoma: Comparison of morbidity and mortality and short-term outcome. *Ann. Surg.* **1999**, *229*, 613–622. [CrossRef] [PubMed]

25. Yeo, C.J.; Cameron, J.L.; Lillemoe, K.D.; Sohn, T.A.; Campbell, K.A.; Sauter, P.K.; Coleman, J.; Abrams, R.A.; Hruban, R.H. Pancreaticoduodenectomy with or without distal gastrectomy and extended retroperitoneal lymphadenectomy for periampullary adenocarcinoma, part 2: Randomized controlled trial evaluating survival, morbidity, and mortality. *Ann. Surg.* **2002**, *236*, 355–366. [CrossRef] [PubMed]

26. Tanaka, A.; Ueno, T.; Oka, M.; Suzuki, T. Effect of denervation of the pylorus and transection of the duodenum on acetaminophen absorption in rats; possible mechanism for early delayed gastric emptying after pylorus preserving pancreatoduodenectomy. *Tohoku J. Exp. Med.* **2000**, *192*, 239–247. [CrossRef] [PubMed]

27. Kim, D.K.; Hindenburg, A.A.; Sharma, S.K.; Suk, C.H.; Gress, F.G.; Staszewski, H.; Grendell, J.H.; Reed, W.P. Is pylorospasm a cause of delayed gastric emptying after pylorus-preserving pancreaticoduodenectomy? *Ann. Surg. Oncol.* **2005**, *12*, 222–227. [CrossRef] [PubMed]

28. Kurahara, H.; Shinchi, H.; Maemura, K.; Mataki, Y.; Iino, S.; Sakoda, M.; Ueno, S.; Takao, S.; Natsugoe, S. Delayed gastric emptying after pancreatoduodenectomy. *J. Surg. Res.* **2011**, *171*, 187–192. [CrossRef]

29. Okabayashi, T.; Kobayashi, M.; Nishimori, I.; Sugimoto, T.; Akimori, T.; Namikawa, T.; Okamoto, K.; Onishi, S.; Araki, K. Benefits of early postoperative jejunal feeding in patients undergoing duodenohemipancreatectomy. *World J. Gastroenterol.* **2006**, *7*, 89–93.

30. Tien, Y.W.; Yang, C.Y.; Wu, Y.M.; Hu, R.H.; Lee, P.H. Enteral nutrition and biliopancreatic diversion effectively minimize impacts of gastroparesis after pancreaticoduodenectomy. *J. Gastrointest. Surg.* **2009**, *13*, 929–937. [CrossRef] [PubMed]

31. Mack, L.A.; Kaklamanos, I.G.; Livingstone, A.S.; Levi, J.U.; Robinson, C.; Sleeman, D.; Franceschi, D.; Bathe, O.F. Gastric decompression and enteral feeding through a double-lumen gastrojejunostomy tube improves outcomes after pancreaticoduodenectomy. *Ann. Surg.* **2004**, *240*, 845–851. [CrossRef] [PubMed]

32. Grizas, S.; Gulbinas, A.; Barauskas, G.; Pundzius, J. A comparison of the effectiveness of the early enteral and natural nutrition after pancreaticoduodenectomy. *Medicina* **2008**, *44*, 678–686. [PubMed]

33. Van Berge Henegouwen, M.I.; Akkermans, L.M.; van Gulik, T.M.; Masclee, A.A.; Moojen, T.M.; Obertop, H.; Gouma, D.J. Prospective randomized trial on the effect of cyclic *vs.* continuous enteral nutrition on postoperative gastric function after pylorus-preserving pancreatoduodenectomy. *Ann. Surg.* **1997**, *226*, 677–685. [CrossRef] [PubMed]

34. Gianotti, L.; Braga, M.; Gentilini, O.; Balzano, G.; Zerbi, A.; di Carlo, V. Artificial nutrition after pancreaticoduodenectomy. *Pancreas* **2000**, *21*, 344–351. [CrossRef] [PubMed]

35. Rayar, M.; Sulpice, L.; Meunier, B.; Boudjema, K. Enteral nutrition reduces delayed gastric emptying after standard pancreaticoduodenectomy with child reconstruction. *J. Gastrointest. Surg.* **2012**, *16*, 1004–1011. [CrossRef] [PubMed]

36. Hallay, J.; Micskei, C.; Fülesdi, B.; Kovács, G.; Szentkereszty, Z.; Takács, I.; Sipka, S.; Bodolay, E.; Sápy, P. Use of three lumen catheter facilitates bowel movement after pancreato-duodenectomy. *Hepatogastroenterology* **2008**, *55*, 1099–1102. [PubMed]

37. Martignoni, M.E.; Friess, H.; Sell, F.; Ricken, L.; Shrikhande, S.; Kulli, C.; Büchler, M.W. Enteral nutrition prolongs delayed gastric emptying in patients after Whipple resection. *Am. J. Surg.* **2000**, *180*, 18–23. [CrossRef] [PubMed]

38. Alexakis, N.; Sutton, R.; Neoptolemos, J.P. Surgical treatment of pancreatic fistula. *Dig. Surg.* **2004**, *21*, 262–274. [CrossRef] [PubMed]

39. Bassi, C.; Dervenis, C.; Butturini, G.; Fingerhut, A.; Yeo, C.; Izbicki, J.; Neoptolemos, J.; Sarr, M.; Traverso, W.; Buchler, M.; *et al.* Postoperative pancreatic fistula: An international study group (ISGPF) definition. *Surgery* **2005**, *138*, 8–13. [CrossRef] [PubMed]

40. Okabayashi, T.; Maeda, H.; Nishimori, I.; Sugimoto, T.; Ikeno, T.; Hanazaki, K. Pancreatic fistula formation after pancreaticooduodenectomy; for prevention of this deep surgical site infection after pancreatic surgery. *Hepatogastroenterology* **2009**, *56*, 519–523. [PubMed]

41. Liu, C.; Du, Z.; Lou, C.; Wu, C.; Yuan, Q.; Wang, J.; Shu, G.; Wang, Y. Enteral nutrition is superior to total parenteral nutrition for pancreatic cancer patients who underwent pancreaticoduodenectomy. *Asia Pac. J. Clin. Nutr.* **2011**, *20*, 154–160. [PubMed]

42. Park, J.S.; Chung, H.K.; Hwang, H.K.; Kim, J.K.; Yoon, D.S. Postoperative nutritional effects of early enteral feeding compared with total parental nutrition in pancreaticoduodectomy patients: A prosepective, randomized study. *J. Korean Med. Sci.* **2012**, *27*, 261–267. [CrossRef] [PubMed]

43. Barlow, R.; Price, P.; Reid, T.D.; Hunt, S.; Clark, G.W.; Havard, T.J.; Puntis, M.C.; Lewis, W.G. Prospective multicentre randomised controlled trial of early enteral nutrition for patients undergoing major upper gastrointestinal surgical resection. *Clin. Nutr.* **2011**, *30*, 560–566. [CrossRef] [PubMed]

44. Wente, M.N.; Veit, J.A.; Bassi, C.; Dervenis, C.; Fingerhut, A.; Gouma, D.J.; Izbicki, J.R.; Neoptolemos, J.P.; Padbury, R.T.; Sarr, M.G.; *et al.* Postpancreatectomy hemorrhage (PPH): An International Study Group of Pancreatic Surgery (ISGPS) definition. *Surgery* **2007**, *142*, 20–25. [CrossRef] [PubMed]

45. Ricci, C.; Casadei, R.; Buscemi, S.; Minni, F. Late postpancreatectomy hemorrhage after pancreaticoduodenectomy: Is it possible to recognize risk factors? *J. Pancreas* **2012**, *13*, 193–198.

46. Gerritsen, A.; Besselink, M.G.; Cieslak, K.P.; Vriens, M.R.; Steenhagen, E.; van Hillegersberg, R.; Borel Rinkes, I.H.; Molenaar, I.Q. Efficacy and complications of nasojejunal, jejunostomy and parenteral feeding after pancreaticoduodenectomy. *J. Gastrointest. Surg.* **2012**, *16*, 1144–1151. [CrossRef] [PubMed]

47. Zhu, X.H.; Wu, Y.F.; Qiu, Y.D.; Jiang, C.P.; Ding, Y.T. Effect of early enteral combined with parenteral nutrition in patients undergoing pancreaticoduodenectomy. *World J. Gastroenterol.* **2013**, *19*, 5889–5896. [CrossRef] [PubMed]

48. Gerritsen, A.; Besselink, M.G.; Gouma, D.J.; Steenhagen, E.; Borel Rinkes, I.H.; Molenaar, I.Q. Systematic review of five feeding routes after pancreatoduodenectomy. *Br. J. Surg.* **2013**, *100*, 589–598. [CrossRef] [PubMed]

49. Yermilov, I.; Jain, S.; Sekeris, E.; Bentrem, D.J.; Hines, O.J.; Reber, H.A.; Ko, C.Y.; Tomlinson, J.S. Utilization of parenteral nutrition following pancreaticoduodenectomy: Is routine jejunostomy tube placement warranted? *Dig. Dis. Sci.* **2009**, *54*, 1582–1588. [CrossRef] [PubMed]

50. Ypsilantis, E.; Praseedom, R.K. Current status of fast-track recovery pathways in pancreatic surgery. *J. Pancreas* **2009**, *10*, 646–650.

51. Braunschweig, C.L.; Levy, P.; Sheean, P.M.; Wang, X. Enteral compared with parenteral nutrition: A meta-analysis. *Am. J. Clin. Nutr.* **2001**, *74*, 534–542. [PubMed]

52. Lewis, S.J.; Egger, M.; Sylvester, P.A.; Thomas, S. Early enteral feeding *vs.* "nil by mouth" after gastrointestinal surgery: Systematic review and meta-analysis of controlled trials. *BMJ* **2001**, *323*, 773–776. [CrossRef] [PubMed]

53. Li, J.; Kudsk, K.A.; Gocinski, B.; Dent, D.; Glezer, J.; Langkamp-Henken, B. Effects of parenteral and enteral nutrition on gut-associated lymphoid tissue. *J. Trauma.* **1995**, *39*, 44–51. [CrossRef] [PubMed]

54. King, B.K.; Kudsk, K.A.; Li, J.; Wu, Y.; Renegar, K.B. Route and type of nutrition influence mucosal immunity to bacterial pneumonia. *Ann. Surg.* **1999**, *229*, 272–278. [CrossRef] [PubMed]

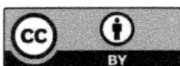

nutrients

MDPI

Article

A Comparison of Postoperative Early Enteral Nutrition with Delayed Enteral Nutrition in Patients with Esophageal Cancer

Gongchao Wang [1,2,†,*], Hongbo Chen [1,†], Jun Liu [1,†], Yongchen Ma [3] and Haiyong Jia [4]

[1] School of Nursing, Shandong University, 44 Wenhua West Road, Jinan 250012, China;
dabo1988@126.com (H.C.); liujunangel@163.com (J.L.)
[2] Thoracic Surgery of Shandong Provincial Hospital, Shandong University, 9677 Jingshi Road,
Jinan 250014, China
[3] School of Medicine, Shandong University, 44 Wenhua West Road, Jinan 250012, China;
myc88587479@hotmail.com
[4] Department of Medicinal Chemistry, Key Laboratory of Chemical Biology (Ministry of Education),
School of Pharmaceutica Sciences, Shandong University, 44 Wenhua West Road, Jinan 250012, China;
502378774@163.com
* Author to whom correspondence should be addressed; wanggongchao@126.com; Tel.: +86-151-6886-3772.
† These authors contributed equally to this work.

Received: 5 May 2015; Accepted: 21 May 2015; Published: 2 June 2015

Abstract: We examined esophageal cancer patients who received enteral nutrition (EN) to evaluate the validity of early EN compared to delayed EN, and to determine the appropriate time to start EN. A total of 208 esophagectomy patients who received EN postoperatively were divided into three groups (Group 1, 2 and 3) based on whether they received EN within 48 h, 48 h–72 h or more than 72 h, respectively. The postoperative complications, length of hospital stay (LOH), days for first fecal passage, cost of hospitalization, and the difference in serum albumin values between pre-operation and post-operation were all recorded. The statistical analyses were performed using the t-test, the Mann-Whitney U test and the chi square test. Statistical significance was defined as $p < 0.05$. Group 1 had the lowest thoracic drainage volume, the earliest first fecal passage, and the lowest LOH and hospitalization expenses of the three groups. The incidence of pneumonia was by far the highest in Group 3 ($p = 0.019$). Finally, all the postoperative outcomes of nutritional conditions were the worst by a significant margin in Group 3. It is therefore safe and valid to start early enteral nutrition within 48 h for postoperative esophageal cancer patients.

Keywords: early enteral nutrition; delayed enteral nutrition; esophageal cancer; postoperative complication

1. Introduction

Esophageal cancer is one of the common malignant tumors in the upper digestive system, which is currently listed as the world's ninth most serious malignant disease [1–3]. Although curative surgery, radiotherapy and chemotherapy improve survival, the five-year survival rate of patients with esophageal cancer is still less than 50% [4]. Factors, such as preoperative diet restrictions, difficulty swallowing and the highly invasive nature of the treatment, cause patients to be prone to malnutrition after esophagectomy [5,6]. During the period that patients cannot take enough food orally, nutrient support plays an important role [7–10]. Nutrition support can be divided into parenteral nutrition and enteral nutrition. As complications of parenteral nutrition are more serious than those of enteral nutrition [11], thoracic surgery doctors use enteral nutrition as the main method of nutrition support. Past studies show that compared with those administered total parental nutrition, early postoperative total enteral nutrition (TEN) in high-risk surgical patients could reduce septic morbidity rates (TPN) [12–15]. Another study indicated that initiating enteral nutrition (EN) within 24 h had no advantage for the postoperative course of the patients with esophageal cancer compared with starting EN at 24–72 h [16]. For early enteral nutrition, opinions vary widely on the extent to which enteral nutrition should begin early. The term "early" was defined as EN started within three days after surgery [17]; however, more recently, "early" has been defined as EN started within 48 or 24 h after surgery [18]. The validity and safety of early EN after esophagectomy has remained controversial [7,16,19]. The aim of the present study is to verify the effectiveness and safety of early EN for the postoperative course and to determine an appropriate time to start enteral nutrition.

2. Patients and Methods

2.1. Patient Selection

Study subjects were selected from patients with esophageal cancer who were admitted for thoracic surgery in the Shandong provincial hospital, affiliated with Shandong University, between January 2013 and October 2014. The study protocol was approved by the Shandong university school of nursing science research project ethics committee (approval number 2012796). Esophageal cancer was diagnosed by gastroscopy. Patients suffering from diabetes or underlying cardiopulmonary diseases, whose body weight loss was more than 10% of the original, were excluded. All patients included in the study did not receive preoperative chemoradiotherapy. Moreover, the patients whose tumor staging was Stage IV (the cancer had spread to other parts of the body) were also excluded because they had lost the chance for curative surgery [20]. All patients received thoracotomy and extensive lymph node dissection during surgery. More specifically, the dissected lymph node included groups 2, 4, 7, 8, 9, 10 on the right side and groups 5, 6, 7, 8, 9, 10 on the left side. Mediastinal lymph node grouping was established according to the International Association for the Study of Lung Cancer (IASLC2009). A total of 208 patients were enrolled in the study. A total of 101 patients in the eastward department of thoracic surgery who received postoperative enteral nutrition within 48 h were included in Group 1. A total of 87 patients in the westward department who received postoperative enteral nutrition within 48–72 h were included in Group 2. For the patients of the two wards, who received early EN and who received very early EN was randomly determined. Twenty patients were included in Group 3 who suffered diarrhea, vomiting or had other adverse reactions after receiving early postoperative enteral nutrition who received enteral nutrition after 72 h.

2.2. Methods

The postoperative patients were given peripheral intravenous nutrition support before EN. Then the Enteral Nutritional Emulsion (TPF-T) (500 mL bag^{-1}) made by Sino-Swed Pharmaceutical Corp. Ltd was used as the nutrition solution for enteral nutrition. The TPF-T was given by nutrition pump uniformly at the same temperature and speed through a nasojejunal tube, which was placed in the jejunum during the operation. The Fat Emulsion, Amino Acids (17) and Glucose (1%) Injection (1440 mL bag^{-1}) made by Sino-Swed Pharmaceutical Corp. Ltd was used as the parenteral nutrition injected by central venous indwelling catheter.

The day before received enteral nutrition, patients were given 150–200 mL 5% glucose and sodium chloride pumping at a speed of 20–25 mL h^{-1}. At the same time, researchers observed the reaction of the patients. If there were no adverse reactions, such as abdominal distention, nausea, or vomiting, the nutrient solution would be started the next day. The total daily calories for all the patients should reach 125.52 kJ (30 kcal) kg^{-1} [21], and insufficient energy would be supplied by parenteral nutrition. On the first day of EN, the patients would be given a total of 500 mL nutrient solution, at a speed of 20–25 mL h^{-1}. The EN dose was increased 500 mL every 24 h if there were no problems related to EN, and reached a maximum dose of 1500 mL every day. The patients (Group 3) who could not tolerate early enteral nutrition were given postoperative enteral nutrition after 72 h. Peripheral intravenous infusions of 5% glucose with electrolyte solutions were also performed to supply water and electrolytes in the three groups. EN continued until the anastomotic healing was confirmed by upper gastrointestinal barium, which would usually be done on the seventh postoperative day [22]. If one developed anastomotic leakage, the amount of time the patient received EN would be extended.

2.3. Clinical Assessment

Clinical factors included age, sex, tumor stage according to the tumor-node-metastasis classification of the International Union against Cancer (7th edition) [20], pathological type, tumor location, surgical stress expressed by operation time (min) and blood loss during surgery (mL). Length of hospital stay (LOH), bowel movement recovery expressed as days for first fecal passage, cost of hospitalization, thoracic drainage volume(mL) were also recorded. The difference of albumin (g L^{-1}) (Δalbumin), total protein (g L^{-1}) (Δtotal protein) and absolute value of lymphocyte ($\times 10^9$ L^{-1}) (Δlymphocyte) between postoperative day 3 and pre-operation, and the difference in weight (Δ' weight), albumin (g L^{-1}) (Δ' albumin), total protein (g L^{-1}) (Δ' total protein) and absolute value of lymphocytes ($\times 10^9$ L^{-1}) (Δ' lymphocyte) between postoperative day 7 and pre-operation were important outcome indicators. Postoperative complications including infectious and noninfectious complications and mortality were also recorded. The infectious complications were those accompanying infections, such as pneumonia or wound infection, and the non-infectious complications were those such as anastomotic fistula or arrhythmia.

2.4. Statistical Analysis

The statistical analyses were performed using the Mann-Whitney U test and adjusted chi-square test. The exact chi-square test was also used if individual cell size was less than 5 counts. The statistical significance was defined as $p < 0.05$. The quantitative data of normality underwent variance analysis and the quantitative data that did not meet normality criteria were analyzed using the rank sum test. Qualitative data were analyzed using the chi-square test. When multiple comparisons were needed, the rank sum test and the chi-square test inspection levels would correct to 0.0125 (0.05/4 = 0.0125) [23].

3. Results

3.1. Pre- and Peri-Operative Clinical Features

Among the 208 patients, 101 patients were categorized into Group 1, 87 patients were categorized into Group 2 and 20 patients were categorized into Group 3. There was no significant difference in mean age, sex, tumor stage, pathological type, tumor location, surgical stress expressed by operation time and blood loss, preoperative nutritional conditions expressed by body weight, or serum total protein values among the three groups. However, serum albumin values were significantly lower in Group 2 of the three groups ($p = 0.001$). Preoperative immune conditions expressed by the absolute value of lymphocyte were also comparable among the groups (Table 1).

Table 1. Pre- and peri-operative clinical features among the three groups.

	Group1 (*n* = 101)	Group2 (*n* = 87)	Group3 (*n* = 20)	*p* value (One-way ANOVA)
Age (years) [a]	58.6 ± 7.5	59.5 ± 8.4	60.3 ± 9.7	0.602
Body weight (kg) [a]	65.2 ± 9.9	64.5 ± 10.4	64.7 ± 6.3	0.89
Operative time (min) [a]	212.7 ± 27.2	204.8 ± 20.0	213.3 ± 34.7	0.083
Blood loss (mL)[a]	213.6 ± 21.9	206.7 ± 17.9	214.5 ± 26.7	0.055
Albumin (g L^{-1}) [a]	42.3 ± 4.7	40.6 ± 3.7	44.2 ± 3.4	0.001
Total protein (g L^{-1}) [a]	69.6 ± 5.4	68.0 ± 5.0	69.9 ± 4.9	0.086
Absolute value of lymphocyte ($\times 10^9$ L^{-1}) [a]	1.89 ± 0.51	1.85 ± 0.48	1.86 ± 0.32	0.808
				p value (Chi square test)
Sex				0.509
Male	90	77	16	
Female	11	10	4	
Stage				0.998
0~IIB	60	52	12	
III	41	35	8	
Pathological type				0.125
Adenocarcinoma	4	0	1	
squamous carcinoma	97	87	19	
	Group1 (*n* = 101)	Group2 (*n* = 87)	Group3 (*n* = 20)	*p* value (Chi square test)
Tumor location				0.173
upper thoracic portion	30	23	2	
mid-thoracic portion	36	42	10	
lower thoracic portion	35	22	8	

[a] Data and mean ± standard deviation.

3.2. Postoperative Complications and Mortality

Postoperative complications were observed in 116 patients (55.77%) and there was a significant difference in whole complications among the three groups (*p* = 0.01). Using a partition of the chi-square method to do multiple comparisons, the result showed that there was a significant difference between Group 1 and Group 3 (*p* = 0.006 < 0.0125). Furthermore, postoperative complications were categorized into two groups: infectious and non-infectious. There was significant difference in the frequency of infectious complications; they were observed most frequently in Group 3 (*p* = 0.008). The frequency of pneumonia observed in the present study was significantly higher in Group 3 out of the three groups (*p* = 0.019). Using a partition of the chi-square method to do multiple comparisons, we found that the difference was rooted in Group 1 and Group 3 (infectious: *p* = 0.003 < 0.0125; pneumonia: *p* = 0.008 < 0.0125). On the other hand, there was no significant difference in non-infectious complications, including anastomotic fistula (*p* = 0.801) and arrhythmia(*p* = 0.353). Perioperative death was observed in only one patient in Group 3. The mortality among the three groups was comparable (*p* = 0.096) (Tables 2 and 3).

Table 2. Postoperative complications and mortality.

	Group1 (*n* = 101)	Group2 (*n* = 87)	Group3 (*n* = 20)	*p* value
Postoperative complications	47	53	16	0.01
Infectious	39	44	15	0.008
Pneumonia	38	43	14	0.019
Wound infection	2	1	1	0.527
Non-infectious	11	15	4	0.353
Anastomotic fistula	6	6	2	0.801
Arrhythmia	5	9	2	0.353
Mortality	0	0	1	0.096

Table 3. Multiple comparison among groups (*p* value).

		Pneumonia (*p* value)	Infectious (*p* value)	Postoperative complications (*p* value)
Group1	Group2	0.103	0.1	0.049
	Group3	0.008	0.003	0.006
Group2	Group3	0.096	0.048	0.108

$\alpha' = 0.05/4 = 0.0125$.

3.3. Postoperative Outcomes Among Group1, Group2 and Group3

There was a significant difference in the indicators of nutritional conditions including Δ' weight, Δalbumin, Δtotal protein, Δ' albumin, and Δ' total protein among the three groups (Table 4). The results of further multiple comparisons showed that all the outcomes of nutritional conditions were the highest in Group 3 of the three groups and there was no significant difference between Group 1 and Group 2 except Δ' albumin (5.79 *vs.* 7.62; *p* = 0.01) (Table 5). Δlymphocyte and Δ lymphocyte that showed the immune conditions of three groups were comparable (*p* = 0.245; *p* = 0.744). There was a significant difference among the three groups in thoracic drainage volume (*p* = 0.004). The results of further multiple comparisons indicated that the thoracic drainage volume in Group 1 was the lowest of the three groups (Group 1 *vs.* Group 2, *p* = 0.008; Group 1 *vs.* Group 3, *p* = 0.009). However, the volumes in Group 2 and Group 3 were comparable (*p* = 0.195). The first fecal passage was observed the earliest in Group 1 and latest in Group 3. LOH and hospitalization expenses were the lowest in Group 1 and the highest in Group 3.

Table 4. Postoperative outcomes among 3 groups.

	Group 1	Group 2	Group 3	*p* value
Δ' weight (kg) [b]	1 ± 2	1 ± 3	5 ± 3	0.000
Thoracic drainage volume (mL) [b]	680 ± 562.5	920 ± 571.25	1065 ± 737.5	0.004
First fecal passage (day) [a]	4.03 ± 0.71	4.93 ± 0.85	6.5 ± 0.95	0.000
LOH (day) [a]	20.82 ± 3.91	23.85 ± 7.80	26.80 ± 5.11	0.000
Hospitalization expenses (yuan) [a]	48,658.71 ± 4823.95	63,218.60 ± 16299.913	76972 ± 7132.38	0.000
Δalbumin (g L^{-1}) [a]	9.88 ± 5.01	10.30 ± 4.54	13.75 ± 5.36	0.006
Δtotal protein (g L^{-1}) [a]	13.01 ± 6.05	14.55 ± 6.62	19.46 ± 8.70	0.000
Δlymphocyte ($\times 10^9$ L^{-1}) [a]	1.02 ± 0.44	0.99 ± 0.45	0.83 ± 0.35	0.245
Δ' albumin (g L^{-1}) [a]	5.79 ± 4.77	7.62 ± 5.05	10.74 ± 4.32	0.000
Δ' total protein (g L^{-1}) [a]	6.44 ± 6.04	7.05 ± 6.93	10.72 ± 6.11	0.027
Δ' lymphocyte ($\times 10^9$ L^{-1}) [a]	0.50 ± 0.47	0.53 ± 0.46	0.57 ± 0.34	0.744

[a] Data and mean ± standard deviation; [b] Median ± range interquartile; Δ: the difference between day 3 and pre-operation; Δ': the difference between day 7 and pre-operation; LOH: length of hospital stay.

4. Discussion

As the results showed in the baseline level of patients, aside from the preoperative albumin levels among the groups having a significant difference (*P* = 0.001, Group 1 = 42.3g L^{-1}, Group 2 = 40.6 g L^{-1}, Group 3 = 44.2 g L^{-1}), there was no significant difference in the general situation of the patients, such as age, gender, pathological type, tumor location, tumor staging and the indexes reflecting the immune condition of nutrition. Surgical stress expressed by operation time and blood loss was also comparable among the three groups. However, the present study was a quasi-experimental research, and the differences before and after the operation were the key point rather than the absolute values. Therefore, the influence of the inconsistency of preoperative baseline levels on the results was small.

Table 5. The results of the multiple comparison (*p* value).

		Δweight (kg)	Thoracic drainage volume (mL)	First fecal passage (day)	LOH (day)	Hospitalization expenses (yuan)
Group1	Group2	0.483	0.008	0.000	0.001	0.000
	Group3	0.000	0.009	0.000	0.000	0.000
Group2	Group3	0.000	0.195	0.000	0.047	0.000
		Δ albumin (g L^{-1})	Δtotal protein (g L^{-1})	Δ′ albumin (g L^{-1})	Δ′ total protein (g L^{-1})	–
Group1	Group2	0.562	0.113	0.01	0.522	–
	Group3	0.001	0.000	0.000	0.007	–
Group2	Group3	0.005	0.003	0.01	0.022	–

$$\alpha' = 0.05/4 = 0.0125.$$

The postoperative complications included pulmonary infection (45.67%), incision infection (1.92%), anastomotic fistula (6.73%) and arrhythmia (7.69%). Atrial fibrillation was the most common arrhythmia. There was a significant difference among the groups in terms of pulmonary infection ($p = 0.019 < 0.05$), and the multiple comparison showed that statistical differences existed between Group 1 and Group 3 ($p = 0.008 < 0.0125$, Group 1 = 80.85%, Group 3 = 87.5%). There was no significant difference among groups in the other three kinds of complications. The results were inconsistent with those of Kazuaki Kobayashi *et al.* [7]. In the research of Kazuaki Kobayashi, there was only a difference in the incidence of anastomotic dehiscence ($p < 0.01$, Group E = 33.33%; Group L = 9.84%) between the two groups and the incidence of pulmonary infection did not differ between the two groups ($p > 0.05$, Group E = 16.67%; Group L = 16.39%). The author gave the following explanation: "A possible explanation for this was that the patients in Group E received damage by preoperative chemotherapy, which was more frequently observed in Group E compared with Group L. The damage to cell recycling, vascularization, and tissue regeneration may affect the anastomotic failure, which was more frequent in Group E." The patients in this study did not receive preoperative systemic chemotherapy and radiotherapy, so there was no difference in this aspect among the groups. Inconsistent results for the incidence of pulmonary infection of the two studies may be associated with the different grouping of the two studies. In Kazuaki Kobayashi's study, the patients were divided into two groups: Group E contained the patients who received EN by postoperative day 3, and Group L contained the patients who received EN after postoperative day 3. However, the present study included three groups: postoperative EN started within 48 h, 48–72 h or after 72 h. The difference of the incidence of the pulmonary infection among the groups existed between Group 1 (within 48 h) and Group 3 (after 72 h). In other words, the incidence of the pulmonary infection of Group 1 was greater than that of Group 3. Consequently, the earlier enteral nutrition began, the lower the incidence of pulmonary infection would be. Moreover, decrease of incidence of pulmonary infection could not only reduce the use of antibiotics after operation, but could also shorten the duration of hospitalization and reduce its cost [24].

Beyond that, there were significant differences in the indicators of nutritional conditions including deviations in weight, albumin and total protein preoperatively and postoperatively among the three groups. The results of further multiple comparisons showed that statistical differences existed between Group 1 and Group 3 as well as Group 2 and Group 3, but no significant difference existed between Group 1 and Group 2 in all the outcomes of nutritional conditions except the difference in serum albumin values between day 7 and pre-operation (Δ′ albumin). In other words, the results of the two early enteral nutrition groups (Group 1 and Group 2) were better than the delayed enteral nutrition group (Group 3), but there was no significant difference between the two early enteral nutrition groups. A possible explanation for this is as follows: (1) For the outcomes used to describe the difference between day 3 and pre-operation, comparison among the three groups was equivalent to the comparison between enteral nutrition and parenteral nutrition because the patients of Group 3 received parenteral nutrition within three days after the operation. Parenteral nutrition simply led to the recovery of patients of Group 3 slower than that of patients of Group 1 and Group 2 [9]. (2) For the outcomes used to describe the difference between day 7 and pre-operation, the nutritional status of the

Nutrients **2015**, *7*, 4308–4317

patients in Group 3 was still worse than the patients in Group 1 and Group 2 due to the delayed start time of enteral nutrition. (3) Considering difference in the start time of enteral nutrition for Group 1 and Group 2 was only about 24 h, the indicators of nutritional conditions were not very sensitive. Consequently, there was no significant difference between Group 1 and Group 2. Moreover, the results of further multiple comparisons of first fecal passage, LOH and hospitalization expenses showed that there was significant difference in the any two groups of the three groups. More specifically, the results of Group 1 were the best of the three groups: the time for first fecal passage was the earliest, LOH was the shortest and the hospitalization expenses were the lowest. Group 2 ranked second and Group 3 ranked the last. Thus, it could be seen that the earlier enteral nutrition started, the faster gastrointestinal function recovered. Moreover, one of the factors affecting hospitalization expenses was hospitalization time. The longer the length of time, the higher the expenses, so there was an inherent relationship between the two outcomes.

In summary, if the patients can adapt well, enteral nutrition should be started within 48 h after the operation. There are three reasons for this: (1) Although there was no significant difference between Group 1 and Group 2 in the indicators of nutritional conditions, the time for first fecal passage was earlier in Group 1, which showed that early enteral nutrition could promote intestinal function recovery. As the view that as long as intestines are functioning, we should use enteral nutrition has become popular in China, we should start enteral nutrition as early as possible. (2) Considering the economic perspective, the cost of enteral nutrition liquid was less than the parenteral nutrition solution, so enteral nutrition should be started as early as possible in order to reduce the economic burden of patients. (3) The safety coefficient of parenteral nutrition is lower than that of enteral nutrition. Parenteral nutrition easily leads to long-term catheter infection, high nutritional and metabolic disorders and respiratory and intestinal complications for patients [11]. Therefore, considering patient safety, enteral nutrition should be started as early as possible.

Finally, under the conditions of clinical work, the present study was a quasi-experiment. Grouping was not random, so it might have led to the occurrence of bias. Especially, non randomisation of the subjects in Group 3 may affect the validity of the results. It was suggested that the experimental design of future research should be improved. Randomized controlled trials of large samples and multicenter studies are needed to provide reliable evidence for implementing early enteral nutrition safely and effectively.

5. Conclusions

Early enteral nutrition within 48 h is safe and valid for postoperative esophageal cancer patients and has advantages in reducing the incidence of postoperative pulmonary infection, improving postoperative nutrition status, promoting early recovery of intestinal movement, shortening hospitalization time and reducing the cost of hospitalization.

Author Contributions: G.W., H.C. and J.L. designed the study; H.C. and J.L. collected the data; J.L. and H.J. entered the data; H.C. and J.L. drafted the manuscript; H.C. and Y.M. undertook the statistical analysis; All authors read and approved the final manuscript.

Conflicts of Interest: The authors declare no conflicts of interest.

References

1. Chen, W.; He, Y.; Zheng, R.; Zhang, S.; Zeng, H.; Zou, X.; He, J. Esophageal cancer incidence and mortality in China, 2009. *J. Thorac. Dis.* **2013**, *5*, 19–26. [PubMed]

2. Huang, Y.M.; Quan, L.L.; Li, Y. Esophageal surgery perioperative nursing. *J. Heilongjiang Med.* **2013**, *6*, 1174–1178.

3. Cho, J.W.; Choi, S.C.; Jang, J.Y.; Shin, S.K.; Choi, K.D.; Lee, J.H.; Kim, S.G.; Sung, J.K.; Jeon, S.W.; Choi, L.J.; *et al.* Lymph Node Metastases in Esophageal Carcinoma: An Endoscopist's View. *J. Clin. Endosc.* **2014**, *47*, 523–529. [CrossRef] [PubMed]

4. Ligthart-Melis, G.C.; Weijs, P.J.M.; Te Boveldt, N.D.; Buskermolen, S.; Earthman, C.P.; Verheul, H.M.W.; de Lange-de Klerk, E.S.M.; van Weyenberg, S.J.B.; van der Peet, D.L. Dietician-delivered intensive nutritional support is associated with a decrease in severe postoperative complications after surgery in patients with esophageal cancer. *J. Dis. Esophagus* **2013**, *26*, 587–593. [CrossRef] [PubMed]
5. Haffejee, A.A.; Angorn, I.B. Nutritional status and the nonspecific cellular and humoral immune response in esophageal carcinoma. *J. Ann. Surg.* **1979**, *189*, 475.
6. Nishi, M.; Hiramatsu, Y.; Hioki, K.; Kojima, Y.; Sanada, T.; Yamanaka, H.; Yamamoto, M. Risk factors in relation to postoperative complications in patients undergoing esophagectomy or gastrectomy for cancer. *J. Ann. Surg.* **1988**, *207*, 148. [CrossRef]
7. Kobayashi, K.; Koyama, Y.; Kosugi, S.; Ishikawa, T.; Sakamoto, K.; Ichikawa, H.; Wakai, T. Is early enteral nutrition better for postoperative course in esophageal cancer patients? *J. Nutr.* **2013**, *5*, 3461–3469. [CrossRef] [PubMed]
8. Smedley, F.; Bowling, T.; James, M.; Stokes, E.; Goodger, C.; O'Ccnnor, O.; Oldale, C.; Jones, P.; Silk, D. Randomized clinical trial of the effects of preoperative and postoperative oral nutritional supplements on clinical course and cost of care. *Br. J. Surg.* **2004**, *91*, 983–990. [CrossRef] [PubMed]
9. Yu, X.B.; Lin, Q.; Qin, X.; Ren, Z.; Zhang, J.; Zhang, J.H.; Zhang, Q.J. Efficacy of early postoperative enteral nutrition in supporting patients after esophagectomy. *Minerva Chir.* **2014**, *69*, 37–46.
10. Fujita, T.; Daiko, H.; Nishimura, M. Early enteral nutrition reduces the rate of life-threatening complications after thoracic esophagectomy in patients with esophageal cancer. *J. Eur. Surg. Res.* **2012**, *48*, 79–84. [CrossRef] [PubMed]
11. Liu, J.C.; Xiong, H.P. *Esophageal Surgery*; Science Press: Beijing, China, 2010; pp. 378–379.
12. Moore, F.A.; Feliciano, D.V.; Andrassy, R.J.; McArdle, R.J.; Booth, F.V.; Morgenstein-Wagner, T.B.; Kellum, J.M.; Welling, R.E.; Moore, E.E. Early enteral feeding, compared with parenteral, reduces postoperative septic complications. The results of a meta-analysis. *J. Ann. Surg.* **1992**, *216*, 172. [CrossRef]
13. Liu, H.S. Research progress of early enteral nutrition in patients with esophageal cancer after operation. *China J. Prac. Nurs.* **2011**, *27*, 77–78.
14. Barlow, R.; Price, P.; Reid, T.D.; Hunt, S.; Clark, G.W.B.; Havard, T.J.; Puntis, M.C.A.; Lewis, W.G. Prospective multicentre randomised controlled trial of early enteral nutrition for patients undergoing major upper gastrointestinal surgical resection. *J. Clin. Nutr.* **2011**, *30*, 560–566. [CrossRef] [PubMed]
15. Zhao, G.; Cao, S.; Zhang, K.; Xin, Y.; Han, J.; Dong, Q.; Cui, J. Effect of early enteral nutrition on immune response and clinical outcomes after esophageal cancer surgery. *J. Chin. Gastrointest. Surg.* **2014**, *17*, 356–360.
16. Manba, N.; Koyama, Y.; Kosugi, S.; Ishikawa, T.; Ichikawa, H.; Minagawa, M.; Kobayashi, T.; Wakai, T. Is early enteral nutrition initiated within 24 hours better for the postoperative course in esophageal cancer surgery? *J. Clin. Med. Res.* **2014**, *6*, 53. [CrossRef] [PubMed]
17. Garrel, D.R.; Davignon, I.; Lopez, D. Length of care in patients with severe burns with or without early enteral nutritional support. A retrospective study. *J. Burn Care Rehab.* **1990**, *12*, 85–90.
18. Doig, G.S.; Heighes, P.T.; Simpson, F.; Sweetman, E.A.; Davies, A.R. Early enteral nutrition, provided within 24 h of injury or intensive care unit admission, significantly reduces mortality in critically ill patients: a meta-analysis of randomised controlled trials. *J. Intensive Care Med.* **2009**, *35*, 2018–2027. [CrossRef] [PubMed]
19. Wheble, G.A.C.; Benson, R.A.; Khan, O.A. Is routine postoperative enteral feeding after oesophagectomy worthwhile? *J. Interact. Cardiovasc. Thorac. Surg.* **2012**, *15*, 709–712. [CrossRef] [PubMed]
20. Sobin, L.H.; Mary, K.; Gospodarowicz, C.W. *TNM Classification of Malignant Tumours*; John Wiley & Sons: Hoboken, NJ, USA, 2011.
21. Hill, G.L.; Church, J. Energy and protein requirements of general surgical patients requiring intravenous nutrition. *Br. J. Surg.* **1984**, *71*, 1–9. [CrossRef] [PubMed]
22. Lai, M.D.; Xu, F.Y. Repair of injury. In *Pathology*, 1st ed.; Sun, B.C., Ed.; Peking University Medical Press: Beijing, China, 2009; pp. 33–34.

Nutrients **2015**, *7*, 4308–4317

23. Benjamini, Y.; Yekutieli, D. The control of the false discovery rate in multiple testing under dependency. *J. Ann. Stat.* **2001**, *29*, 1165–1188.

24. Farran, L.; Llop, J.; Sans, M.; Kreisler, E.; Miro, M.; Galan, M.; Rafecas, A. Efficacy of enteral decontamination in the prevention of anastomotic dehiscence and pulmonary infection in esophagogastric surgery. *J. Dis. Esophagus* **2008**, *21*, 159–164. [CrossRef] [PubMed]

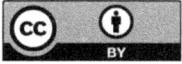

nutrients

MDPI

Article

Enteral Immunomodulatory Diet (Omega-3 Fatty Acid, γ-Linolenic Acid and Antioxidant Supplementation) for Acute Lung Injury and Acute Respiratory Distress Syndrome: An Updated Systematic Review and Meta-Analysis

Congcong Li †, Liyan Bo †, Wei Liu, Xi Lu * and Faguang Jin *

Department of Respiratory and Critical Care Medicine, Tangdu Hospital, Fourth Military Medical University, Xinsi Road 1, Xi'an 710038, China; licong1988@hotmail.com (C.L.); boliyan@hotmail.com (L.B.); liuweilung@163.com (W.L.)
* Authors to whom correspondence should be addressed; luxi1126@163.com (X.L.); jinfag@fmmu.edu.cn (F.J.); Tel./Fax: +86-029-84777425.
† These authors contributed equally to this work.

Received: 15 May 2015; Accepted: 23 June 2015; Published: 9 July 2015

Abstract: Enteral immunomodulatory nutrition is considered as a promising therapy for the treatment of acute lung injury and acute respiratory distress syndrome (ALI/ARDS). However, there are still some divergences, and it is unclear whether this treatment should be recommended for patients with ALI/ARDS. Therefore, we conducted this systematic review and meta-analysis to assess the efficacy and safety of an enteral immunomodulatory diet on the clinical outcomes of ALI/ARDS patients. Methods: We retrieved potentially relevant clinical trials though electronic databases. All trials of enteral immunomodulatory diet for ALI/ARDS were included. Analyses of the overall all-cause mortality, 28-day ventilator-free days and 28-day intensive care unit (ICU) free days were conducted. Results: In total six controlled trials were evaluated. The pooled results did not show a significant reduction in the risk of all-cause mortality (M-H RR (the overall Mantel-Haenszel relative risk), 0.81 (95% CI, 0.50–1.31); $p = 0.38$; 6 trials, $n = 717$) in ALI/ARDS patients treated with the immunomodulatory diet. This treatment also did not extend the ventilator-free days and ICU-free days. However, patients with high mortality might benefit from this treatment. Conclusions: The enteral immunomodulatory diet could not reduce the severity of the patients with ALI/ARDS. Whereas, for ALI/ARDS patients with high mortality, this treatment might reduce the all-cause mortality, but its use should be treated with discretion.

Keywords: enteral nutrition; immunomodulatory diet; acute respiratory distress syndrome; acute lung injury; critical care; mortality

---

1. Introduction

Since its first description in 1967, acute lung injury (ALI) and acute respiratory distress syndrome (ARDS) have been known as common and lethal diseases. With mortality ranging from 25%–40% [1], ALI/ARDS is a life-threatening disorder that cannot be ignored. It is mainly caused by predisposing disorders such as pneumonia, aspiration, shock, and severe sepsis [2]. Benefiting from the exploration of the pathophysiology of ALI/ARDS, we know that after having been affected by these diseases, neutrophils will infiltrate into the alveolar space and pulmonary mesenchyme, where they will release pro-inflammatory cytokines and eventually cause ALI/ARDS [2], which is characteristic of leakage of edema fluid and mismatch of ventilation and perfusion [2,3].

Although we know much about the pathophysiologic change of ALI/ARDS, very little improvement in patient outcomes has been achieved. The main treatment is supportive care, including maintaining oxygenation and avoiding complications [1,2]. There are no specific and effective treatments for ALI/ARDS [4], although many ventilation strategies and medicines have been tried. Thus, it is urgent to find an effective treatment for ALI/ARDS. Over the past two decades, some trials [5–7] and meta-analyses [8,9] have suggested that the enteral use of an immunomodulatory diet (omega-3 fatty acid, γ-linolenic acid and antioxidant supplementation) might be a promising therapy.

This immunomodulatory diet is mainly combined with anti-inflammatory elements (such as eicosapentaenoic acid (EPA), docosahexaenoic acid (DHA) and gamma-linolenic acid (GLA)) and antioxidants (such as vitamin C, vitamin E and beta-carotene). It has been reported that Omega-3 (EPA and DHA) could modulate inflammatory processes, such as by reducing leukotriene production [10,11] and decreasing the synthesis of prostaglandin E2 [12]. It can also reduce the permeability of the alveolar-capillary membrane [13]. As for the antioxidants, they can scavenge free radicals, as we all know, and thus reduce the inflammation [14].

Using enteral nutrition for ALI/ARDS patients has been demonstrated to improve oxygenation and extend 28-day ventilator-free days and 28-day intensive care unit (ICU) free days [5,7]. It has even been associated with reduced mortality [6,7]. Some meta-analyses [8,9] have also shown its effect. However, one trial conducted by Rice *et al.* [15] revealed that an enteral inflammation-modulating diet did not improve the outcomes of ALI/ARDS patients and might be harmful. This conclusion compelled us to re-evaluate the effectiveness and safety of this treatment.

Therefore, we conducted this systematic review and meta-analysis to re-evaluate the effectiveness and safety of enteral use of the immunomodulatory diet (omega-3 fatty acid, γ-linolenic acid and antioxidant supplementation) *vs.* standard enteral nutrition on the mortality and clinical outcomes in patients with ALI/ARDS and to guide further research in this area.

2. Methods

The work, including the literature search, study selection and data extraction, was conducted according to standard strategies described below. Two reviewers (CCL and LYB) completed this work independently, and all discrepancies were solved by discussion or consultation with the senior reviewer (FGJ). Ethical approval was not required to conduct this meta-analysis.

2.1. Search Strategy

An extensive computer search of the relevant literature was performed by the two reviewers independently using databases including MEDLINE (PubMed), Embase and the Cochrane Central Register of Controlled Trials. We also retrieved potentially relevant literature manually, including conference abstracts published in the American Journal of Respiratory and Critical Care Medicine, Critical Care Medicine and Chest. All articles and conference abstracts about enteral nutrition therapies for patients with ALI or ARDS were identified regardless of language. The search terms we used were critically ill patients, acute lung injury, ALI, acute respiratory distress syndrome, ARDS, mechanical ventilation, sepsis, immunomodulatory diet, fish oil, antioxidants, omega-3 fatty acids, eicosapentaenoic acid (EPA), docosahexaenoic acid (DHA) and γ-linolenic acid (GLA).

2.2. Study Selection

Studies were included if they fulfilled all of the inclusion criteria. (1) Participants: patients had to be diagnosed with ALI/ARDS or have respiratory failure that required mechanical ventilation. (2) Type of studies: studies were eligible only if they were randomized controlled trials. (3) Type of interventions: studies used enteral nutrition therapies (omega-3 fatty acids, γ-linolenic acid and antioxidants). Studies were excluded if they did not provide outcomes related to mortality, 28-day ventilator-free days or 28-day ICU-free days. Crossover studies were also excluded.

2.3. End Points and Data Extraction

The primary end point was all-cause mortality, and the secondary end points were 28-day ventilator-free days, 28-day ICU-free days and adverse effects. For all-cause mortality, we used 28-day mortality. If 28-day mortality could not be acquired, we used ICU or hospital mortality instead. We also extracted and collected the relevant information about each study, such as the characteristics of the studies, characteristics of the participants, enteral immunomodulatory therapy strategies and types of outcomes.

2.4. Quality Assessment

The quality levels of the included trials were also evaluated independently by two authors (CCL and LYB). We assessed the risk of bias (including selection bias, performance bias, attrition bias, detection bias, reporting bias and other bias) using the assessment table recommended by the Cochrane Reviewers' Handbook [16]. We also evaluated the methodological quality of the included trials using the Modified Jadad Scale [17], where the full score is 7, and scores of 4–7 are regarded as high quality and 1–3 as low quality.

2.5. Data Processing and Statistical Analysis

First, we examine the heterogeneity of the included studies using the I^2 statistic and Chi^2 test, with significant heterogeneity if $p \leq 0.10$ for the Chi^2 test or $I^2 \geq 50\%$. If significant heterogeneity was obtained, we would use the random-effects model for the following analysis; otherwise, the fixed-effects model would be used.

Second, we pooled the treatment effects of enteral nutrition on the all-cause mortality to estimate the summary effect. As the mortality outcome was dichotomous, we calculated the relative risk (RR) and 95% confidence interval (CI) of every included trial and then pooled them to estimate the overall Mantel-Haenszel (M-H) RR and the 95% CI. For the continuous variables, we calculated the standardized mean difference (SMD). To test the robustness of the results, we performed a sensitivity analysis by excluding each individual study and re-analyzing. The funnel plot was calculated to evaluate the publication bias.

The results were considered statistically significant if (1) the two-sided p-value ≤ 0.05, (2) the confidence interval for RR did not include 1, and (3) the confidence interval for SMD did not include 0. The data synthesis and sensitivity analyses were performed using Review Manager (version 5.1).

3. Results

3.1. Study Selection and Quality Assessment

We identified six studies [5–7,15,18,19] that fulfilled our inclusion criteria out of 2274 potential articles though searching the relevant databases (see Figure 1). All of them were included in our analysis. Five relevant papers [20–24] were excluded based on the reasons described in Table S1. The major characteristics of the six included trials are summarized in Table 1. In short, the trials encompassed a total of 717 patients, with 365 patients in the experimental groups and 352 patients in the control groups. The mean age of the patients ranged from 51.0 to 65.1. The mortality of the control groups ranged from 12.5% to 57.14%. When stratified by the compositions of the immunomodulatory diet, two studies included treatment with EPA + GLA + antioxidants, and four studies included treatment with EPA + DHA + GLA + antioxidants. When stratified by the blind strategies, four trials were double-blind, one trial was single-blind and one trial was unblinded.

We evaluated the quality of the included trials using the Modified Jadad Scale and Cochrane's risk of bias assessment table. As shown in Table S2, all of the included studies were high quality, and most of them had low risk of bias in the generation of random sequence, allocation concealment, incomplete outcome data and selective reporting. Only two trials were high risk in terms of the blinding of participants and personnel.

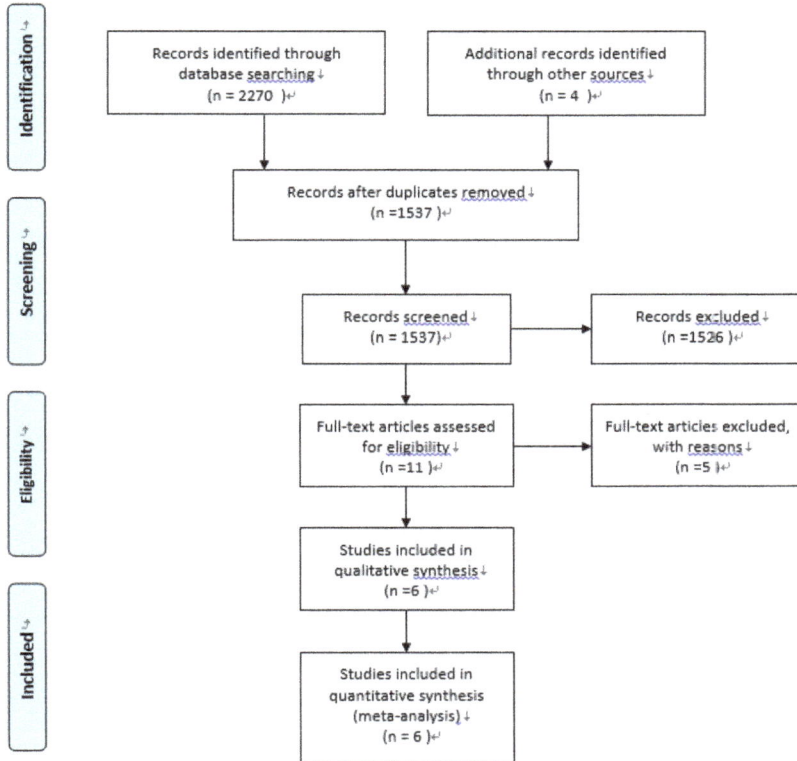

Figure 1. Preferred Reporting Items for Systematic Reviews and Meta-Analyses (PRISMA) Flow Diagram.

Table 1. Characteristics of Included Trials.

Parameter	Gadek et al., 1999	Singe et al., 2006	Pontes-Arda et al., 2006	Grau-Carmona et al., 2011	Rice et al., 2011	Elamin et al., 2012
Interventions	EPA + GLA + antioxidants	EPA + GLA + antioxidants	EPA + DHA + GLA + antioxidants	EPA + DHA + GLA + antioxidants	EPA + DHA + GLA + antioxidants	EPA + DHA + GLA + antioxidants
Control Diet	Isonitrogenous and isocaloric control diet	Isonitrogenous and isocaloric control diet	Isonitrogenous and isocaloric control diet	Isocaloric control diet	Isocaloric and isovolemic control diet	Isonitrogenous and isocaloric control diet
Treatment Duration	N/A	14 days	N/A	N/A	21 days	7 days
Route	Gastric, duodenal, jejunalfeeding tube	Nasogastric, duodenal, jejunal tube	Eneral feeding	Gastric, jejunal tube	Bolus delivery	Nasogastric, nasoduodenal, nasojejunal, jejunostomytubes
Sample Size						
Treatment Group	51	46	55	61	143	9
Control Group	47	49	48	71	129	8
Sex Ratio (Male:Female)	52:46	NA	61:42	30:132	133:139	8:9
Average Age (years)	51	59.7	65.1	63	54.1	52.4
No. of Participants Drop-out or Withdrawal	48	5	62	28	0	5
Blind Type	Double-blind	Unblind	Double-blind	Single-blind	Double-blind	Double-blind
Modified Jadad Scale	7	5	5	5	7	5
Primary End Point	Time receiving ventilatorysupport	Change in oxygenation and breathing patterns	28-day mortality	New organ dysfunction	Ventilator-free days	Oxygenation and modified Lung Injury Scores
Mortality Outcome Type	Mortality	28-day mortality	28-day mortality	28-day mortality	60-day or hospital mortality	28-day mortality
Mortality						
Treatment Group	6/51	13/46	18/55	11/61	38/143	0/9
Control Group	9/47	28/49	25/48	11/71	21/129	1/8
Mortality Rate of Control Group	9/47 (19.15%)	28/49 (57.14%)	25/48 (52.08)	11/71 (15.49)	21/129 (16.28)	1/8 (12.5)
PaO₂/FiO₂ Ratio (Day 7)						
Treatment Group	N/A	296.5 ± 165.3 (SD)	224.4	217	N/A	178
Control Group	N/A	236.3 ± 79.8 (SD)	150.5	190	N/A	201

Abbreviations: EPA, eicosapentaenoic acid; GLA, gamma-linolenic acid; DHA, docosahexaenoic acid; N/A, not available.

3.2. Effect on Mortality

Because significant heterogeneity was found across the included trials ($\chi^2 = 14.61$, df = 5 ($p = 0.01$); $I^2 = 66\%$), we used the random-effects model to analyze the overall effect of immunomodulatory nutrition on mortality. As shown in Figure 2, there was no significant difference between the two groups (M-H RR, 0.81 (95% CI, 0.50–1.31); $p = 0.38$; six trials, $n = 717$) that is, the pooled result did not showed a significant reduction in the risk of all-cause mortality in ALI/ARDS patients treated with immunomodulatory nutrition. The overall mortality of the six trials was 25.24%, and the mortality of the experimental groups was 23.56% compared with 26.99% for the control groups.

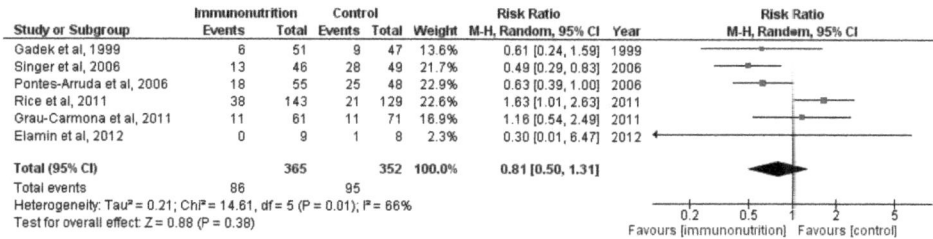

Study or Subgroup	Immunonutrition Events	Total	Control Events	Total	Weight	Risk Ratio M-H, Random, 95% CI	Year	Risk Ratio M-H, Random, 95% CI
Gadek et al, 1999	6	51	9	47	13.6%	0.61 [0.24, 1.59]	1999	
Singer et al, 2006	13	46	28	49	21.7%	0.49 [0.29, 0.83]	2006	
Pontes-Arruda et al, 2006	18	55	25	48	22.9%	0.63 [0.39, 1.00]	2006	
Rice et al, 2011	38	143	21	129	22.6%	1.63 [1.01, 2.63]	2011	
Grau-Carmona et al, 2011	11	61	11	71	16.9%	1.16 [0.54, 2.49]	2011	
Elamin et al, 2012	0	9	1	8	2.3%	0.30 [0.01, 6.47]	2012	
Total (95% CI)		365		352	100.0%	0.81 [0.50, 1.31]		
Total events	86		95					

Heterogeneity: Tau² = 0.21; Chi² = 14.61, df = 5 (P = 0.01); I² = 66%
Test for overall effect: Z = 0.88 (P = 0.38)

Favours [immunonutrition] Favours [control]

Figure 2. Forest plot of the association between enteral immunomodulatory diet and all-cause mortality among patients with ALI (acute lung injury)/ARDS (acute respiratory distress syndrome).

Because of the heterogeneity of the mortality in the control groups across the included trials, we conducted a subgroup analysis by stratifying the previous meta-analyses according to the mortality of the control groups. The analyses (M-H RR, 1.16 (95% CI, 0.70–1.91); $p = 0.56$; three trials, $n = 97$) revealed that for patients with low mortality, this treatment could not reduce the overall mortality in ALI/ARDS patients (see Figure 3). The results (M-H RR, 0.56 (95% CI, 0.40–0.80); $p = 0.001$; two trials, $n = 198$) indicated that patients with high mortality might benefit from this treatment, and there was a significant subgroup difference ($\chi^2 = 5.36$, df = 1 ($p = 0.02$); $I^2 = 81.4\%$). However, they were something that need our attention. The quality of the trials in this subgroup was lower than most of others (as shown in Table S2).

3.3. Effect on 28-Day Ventilator-Free Days and 28-Day ICU-Free Days

We also pooled the data about the 28-day ventilator-free days and 28-day ICU-free days. The outcomes of 568 participants from four trials were available when assessing the effect of enteral nutrition on ventilator-free days and ICU-free days. As shown in Figures 4 and 5, enteral nutrition did not extend the ventilator-free days (M-H RR, −0.33 (95% CI, −0.90–0.24); $p = 0.25$; four trials, $n = 568$) and ICU-free days (M-H RR, −0.30 (95% CI, −0.82–0.22); $p = 0.26$; four trials, $n = 568$). Because of the significant heterogeneity of the included trials (($\chi^2 = 30.79$, df = 3 ($p < 0.00001$); $I^2 = 90\%$) and ($\chi^2 = 25.76$, df = 3 ($p < 0.0001$); $I^2 = 88\%$)), the random-effects model was selected.

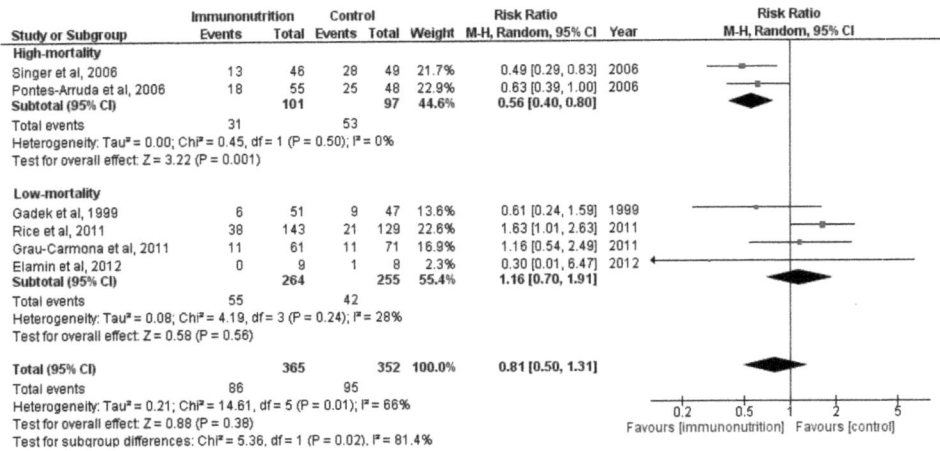

Figure 3. Forest plot of the association between enteral immunomodulatory diet and all-cause mortality among patients with ALI/ARDS, stratified by discrepancy of mortality.

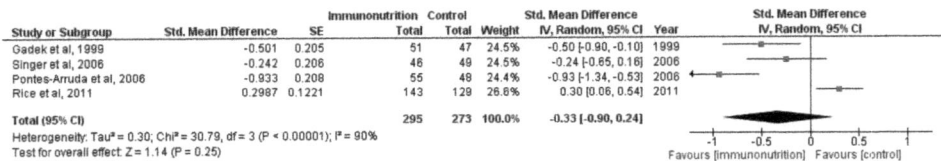

Figure 4. Forest plot of the association between enteral immunomodulatory diet and 28-day ventilator-free days among patients with ALI/ARDS.

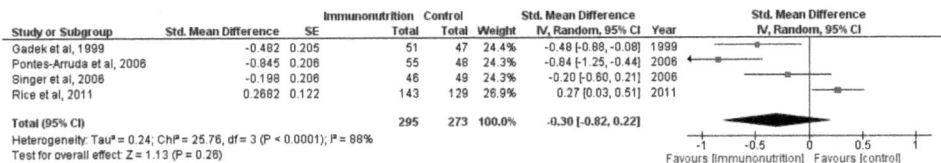

Figure 5. Forest plot of the association between enteral immunomodulatory diet and 28-day ICU-free days among patients with ALI/ARDS.

3.4. Sensitivity Analyses

To test the robustness of the results, we conducted sensitivity analyses. We excluded each individual study, re-analyzing and comparing with the original results. When excluding the trial conducted by Rice T. *et al.* [15], the overall effect was M-H RR, 0.63 (95% CI, 0.47–0.85); $p = 0.0.003$; five trials, $n = 445$ (see Figure S1). When excluding other trials, the results were consistent with the previous one.

3.5. Adverse Effects

To test the safety of this treatment, we also analyzed the adverse effects of the enteral immunomodulatory diet. The majority of adverse events were gastrointestinal events such as diarrhea, dyspepsia and nausea. As shown in Figure 6, there was no significant difference between the two groups (M-H RR, 0.92 (95% CI, 0.57–1.47); *p* =0.72; three trials, *n* =333).

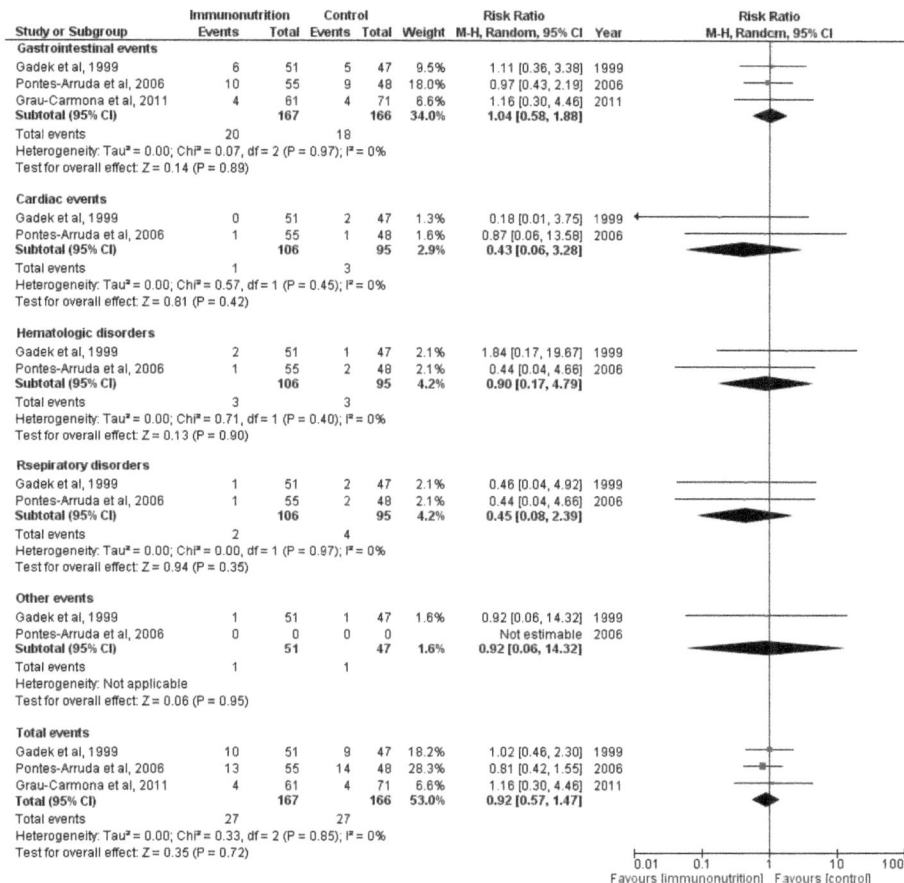

Figure 6. Forest plot of the association between enteral immunomodulatory diet and adverse events among patients with ALI/ARDS.

3.6. Publication Bias

No evidence of publication bias was detected by funnel plots (see Figure S2).

4. Discussion

In conducting this systematic review, we searched the relevant literature comprehensively without language limitation. The pooled results from all six independently conducted trials revealed that an enteral immunomodulatory diet (omega-3 fatty acid, γ-linolenic acid and antioxidant supplementation) could not improve all-cause mortality, ventilator-free days or ICU-free days in patients with ALI/ARDS. Overall, patients could not benefit from enteral immunomodulatory diet, and its use should be treated with discretion.

It was believed previously that the immunomodulatory diet could suppress the elevated inflammatory reactions during ALI/ARDS [5], and patients could benefit from it [6]. Preclinical studies reported that Omega-3 (EPA and DHA) could reduce leukotriene synthesis and the production of prostaglandin E2, which could be beneficial in ALI/ARDS [3,11,13]. The antioxidants could also reduce the inflammation through scavenging free radicals [25]. Several clinical trials confirmed these results [5–7], and demonstrated an association between the usage of enteral immunomodulatory diet and improved outcomes in ALI/ARDS patients [5–7]. Two meta-analyses [8,9] also demonstrated this effect. However, some trials conducted recently achieved a contrary result [15,18], showing that enteral inflammation-modulating diet did not improve the outcomes and might be harmful. Our results were similar. However, some results needed extra attention. As shown in the characteristics of the included studies, the mortality of the control groups varied widely (from 12.50% to 57.14%), and the test for heterogeneity was also significant for mortality. This result may be due to the different severity of the illness and improved treatment strategies [2]. To decrease its influence on the final results, we used the random-effects model for analysis, and we also conducted a subgroup analysis stratified according to the mortality of the control groups. The result revealed that enteral immunomodulatory nutrition could only benefit ALI/ARDS patients with high mortality. For patients with low mortality, this treatment had no effect and might be harmful. From this perspective, it is important to clarify the indications of this treatment, and for future trials about this aspect, the enrolled patients could be restricted to severe cases. However, the quality of the two trials included in the high-mortality subgroup was lower than most of the others, and the results of these studies might be affected.

The drop-out proportions of most included studies were large. Undoubtedly, the reliabilities of the final results achieved by these trials were influenced by this factor [16]. The main reason that people left the studies was that the patients could not tolerate the rate of continuous enteral infusions because of gastrointestinal complications [5,7]. However, the study conducted by Rice T. *et al.* [15] solved this problem by using bolus delivery, namely small-volume supplementation, to deliver the supplements. The results indicated that this method was more tolerable. However, given 120 mL fluid once might increase the risk of aspiration, especially for patients who already have respiratory compromise.

In this review, we demonstrated that ALI/ARDS patients could not benefit from enteral immunomodulatory diet through including some newly reported trials. However, we still need further exploration of the following issues. During sensitivity analyses, we found that the results were not very robust. The final conclusion was seriously affected by the trial conducted by Rice T. *et al.* When we excluded this study, re-analyzed and compared with the previous results, the opposite conclusion was obtained. This condition was more or less due to the discrepancy of the controlled nutrition, and the calorie intake was quite low in Rice T. *et al.*'s trials [26]. However, the reason is still unclear, and we should be aware that the conclusion is not certain. Further improved randomized clinical trials are needed.

Some limitations in this report should be mentioned. First, the heterogeneity tests of the all-cause mortality, ventilator-free days and ICU-free days were positive. Although we tried to reduce their influence methodologically (using a random-effects model and subgroup analyses), they might still cause some biases. Second, the sample sizes of the included trials were small, and only three trials had more than 100 patients available. Even worse, the drop-out proportions were large in the majority of the included trials. Third, there was also some variability in the patient types, outcome types, and route of intervention administration. When trying to solve this problem, we found clues indicating that the effects of enteral nutrition may be related to the severity of the ALI/ARDS. Finally, we did not assess the discrepancy of the ratio of partial pressure arterial oxygen and fraction of inspired oxygen (PaO2/FiO2 ratio) because of inadequate information. As one of the most frequently used indicators of oxygenation and respiratory function, the PaO2/FiO2 ratio is a good predictor of the condition of ALI/ARDS patients. Thus, further trials should report more information about it.

5. Conclusions

Overall, based on the existing data, the enteral immunomodulatory diet (omega-3 fatty acid, γ-linolenic acid and antioxidant supplementation) could not reduce the mortality of patients with

Nutrients **2015**, *7*, 5572–5585

ALI/ARDS and also could not extend the 28-day ventilator-free days or 28-day ICU-free days. However, the subgroup analysis showed that enteral immunomodulatory nutrition could benefit ALI/ARDS patients with high mortality, but it should be used with discretion. More well-designed clinical trials are urgently needed to verify this conclusion.

Appendix Supplementary Information

Table S1: Studies excluded from the meta-analysis of clinical trials involving enteral nutrition treatment for ALI/ARDS.

Table S2: Risk of bias of the included studies.

Figure S1: Sensitivity results (overall effect when excluding the trial conducted by Rice T. *et al.*).

Figure S2: Funnel plot of the standard error by log relative risk of all-cause mortality.

Acknowledgments: The conduct of this study was not funded. The authors thank Anan Yin for his support during revision of this manuscript.

Author Contributions: All authors contributed to the inception of the research question and study design. Congcong Li also contributed to the study selection, quality assessment and manuscript composition. Liyan Bo contributed to the study selection, quality assessment, and records review. Wei Liu and Xi Lu contributed to the data synthesis and data analysis. Faguang Jin and Xi Lu were responsible for the integrity of this work and contributed to the study design, final study selection and manuscript review. All authors contributed to drafting the manuscript and have read and approved the final manuscript.

Conflicts of Interest: The authors declare no conflict of interest.

References

1. Wheeler, A.P.; Bernard, G.R. Acute lung injury and the acute respiratory distress syndrome: A clinical review. *Lancet* **2007**, *369*, 1553–1564. [CrossRef]
2. Pierrakos, C.; Karanikolas, M.; Scolletta, S.; Karamouzos, V.; Velissaris, D. Acute respiratory distress syndrome: Pathophysiology and therapeutic options. *J. Clin. Med. Res.* **2012**, *4*, 7–16. [CrossRef] [PubMed]
3. Muller-Redetzky, H.C.; Felten, M.; Hellwig, K.; Wienhold, S.M.; Naujoks, J.; Opitz, B.; Kershaw, O.; Gruber, A.D.; Suttorp, N.; Witzenrath, M. Increasing the inspiratory time and I:E ratio during mechanical ventilation aggravates ventilator-induced lung injury in mice. *Crit. Care* **2015**, *19*, 23. [CrossRef] [PubMed]
4. Adhikari, N.; Burns, K.E.; Meade, M.O. Pharmacologic treatments for acute respiratory distress syndrome and acute lung injury: Systematic review and meta-analysis. *Treat Respir. Med.* **2004**, *3*, 307–328. [CrossRef] [PubMed]
5. Gadek, J.E.; DeMichele, S.J.; Karlstad, M.D.; Pacht, E.R.; Donahoe, M.; Albertson, T.E.; Van Hoozen, C.; Wennberg, A.K.; Nelson, J.L.; Noursalehi, M. Effect of enteral feeding with eicosapentaenoic acid, gamma-linolenic acid, and antioxidants in patients with acute respiratory distress syndrome. *Crit. Care Med.* **1999**, *27*, 1409–1420. [CrossRef] [PubMed]
6. Singer, P.; Theilla, M.; Fisher, H.; Gibstein, L.; Grozovski, E.; Cohen, J. Benefit of an enteral diet enriched with eicosapentaenoic acid and gamma-linolenic acid in ventilated patients with acute lung injury. *Crit. Care Med.* **2006**, *34*, 1033–1038. [CrossRef] [PubMed]
7. Pontes-Arruda, A.; Aragao, A.M.; Albuquerque, J.D. Effects of enteral feeding with eicosapentaenoic acid, gamma-linolenic acid, and antioxidants in mechanically ventilated patients with severe sepsis and septic shock. *Crit. Care Med.* **2006**, *34*, 2325–2333. [CrossRef] [PubMed]
8. Pontes-Arruda, A.; Demichele, S.; Seth, A.; Singer, P. The use of an inflammation-modulating diet in patients with acute lung injury or acute respiratory distress syndrome: A meta-analysis of outcome data. *JPEN J. Parenter. Enter. Nutr.* **2008**, *32*, 596–605. [CrossRef] [PubMed]
9. Dee, B.M.; Bruno, J.J.; Lal, L.S.; Canada, T.W. Effects of immune-enhancing enteral nutrition on mortality and oxygenation in acute lung injury and acute respiratory distress syndrome a meta-analysis. *Hosp. Pharm.* **2011**, *1*, 33–40. [CrossRef]
10. El, K.D.; Gjorstrup, P.; Filep, J.G. Resolvin E1 promotes phagocytosis-induced neutrophil apoptosis and accelerates resolution of pulmonary inflammation. *Proc. Natl. Acad. Sci. USA* **2012**, *109*, 14983–14988.

11. Khan, S.A.; Ali, A.; Khan, S.A.; Zahran, S.A.; Damanhouri, G.; Azhar, E.; Qadri, I. Unraveling the complex relationship triad between lipids, obesity, and inflammation. *Mediat. Inflamm.* **2014**, *2014*. [CrossRef] [PubMed]

12. Wang, B.; Gong, X.; Wan, J.Y.; Zhang, L.; Zhang, Z.; Li, H.Z.; Min, S. Resolvin D1 protects mice from LPS-induced acute lung injury. *Pulm. Pharmacol. Ther.* **2011**, *24*, 434–441. [CrossRef] [PubMed]

13. Cox, J.R.; Phillips, O.; Fukumoto, J.; Fukumoto, I.; Tamarapu, P.P.; Arias, S.; Cho, Y.; Lockey, R.F.; Kolliputi, N. Aspirin-Triggered Resolvin D1 Treatment Enhances Resolution of Hyperoxic Acute Lung Injury. *Am. J. Respir. Cell Mol. Biol.* **2015**. [CrossRef]

14. Chen, S.; Zheng, S.; Liu, Z.; Tang, C.; Zhao, B.; Du, J.; Jin, H. Endogeous sulfur dioxide protects against oleic acid-induced acute lung injury in association with inhibition of oxidative stress in rats. *Lab. Investig.* **2015**, *95*, 142–156. [CrossRef] [PubMed]

15. Rice, T.W.; Wheeler, A.P.; Thompson, B.T.; DeBoisblanc, B.P.; Steingrub, J.; Rock, P. Enteral omega-3 fatty acid, gamma-linolenic acid, and antioxidant supplementation in acute lung injury. *JAMA* **2011**, *306*, 1574–1581. [CrossRef] [PubMed]

16. Higgins, J.P.; Altman, D.G.; Gotzsche, P.C.; Juni, P.; Moher, D.; Oxman, A.D.; Savovic, J.; Schulz, K.F.; Weeks, L.; Sterne, J.A. The Cochrane Collaboration's tool for assessing risk of bias in randomised trials. *BMJ* **2011**, *343*. [CrossRef] [PubMed]

17. Banares, R.; Albillos, A.; Rincon, D.; Alonso, S.; Gonzalez, M.; Ruiz-del-Arbol, L.; Salcedo, M.; Molinero, L.M. Endoscopic treatment *versus* endoscopic plus pharmacologic treatment for acute variceal bleeding: A meta-analysis. *Hepatology* **2002**, *35*, 609–615. [CrossRef] [PubMed]

18. Grau-Carmona, T.; Moran-Garcia, V.; Garcia-de-Lorenzo, A.; Heras-de-la-Calle, G.; Quesada-Bellver, B.; Lopez-Martinez, J.; Gonzalez-Fernandez, C.; Montejo-Gonzalez, J.C.; Blesa-Malpica, A.; Albert-Bonamusa, I.; *et al.* Effect of an enteral diet enriched with eicosapentaenoic acid, gamma-linolenic acid and anti-oxidants on the outcome of mechanically ventilated, critically ill, septic patients. *Clin. Nutr.* **2011**, *30*, 578–584. [CrossRef] [PubMed]

19. Elamin, E.M.; Miller, A.C.; Ziad, S. Immune enteral nutrition can improve outcomes in medical-surgical patients with ARDS: A prospective randomized controlled trial. *J. Nutr. Disord. Ther.* **2012**, *2*, 109. [CrossRef] [PubMed]

20. Nelson, J.L.; DeMichele, S.J.; Pacht, E.R.; Wennberg, A.K. Effect of enteral feeding with eicosapentaenoic acid, gamma-linolenic acid, and antioxidants on antioxidant status in patients with acute respiratory distress syndrome. *JPEN J. Parenter. Enter. Nutr.* **2003**, *27*, 98–104. [CrossRef]

21. Pacht, E.R.; DeMichele, S.J.; Nelson, J.L.; Hart, J.; Wennberg, A.K.; Gadek, J.E. Enteral nutrition with eicosapentaenoic acid, gamma-linolenic acid, and antioxidants reduces alveolar inflammatory mediators and protein influx in patients with acute respiratory distress syndrome. *Crit. Care Med.* **2003**, *31*, 491–500. [CrossRef] [PubMed]

22. Theilla, M.; Singer, P.; Cohen, J.; Dekeyser, F. A diet enriched in eicosapentanoic acid, gamma-linolenic acid and antioxidants in the prevention of new pressure ulcer formation in critically ill patients with acute lung injury: A randomized, prospective, controlled study. *Clin. Nutr.* **2007**, *26*, 752–757. [CrossRef] [PubMed]

23. Pontes-Arruda, A.; Martins, L.F.; de Lima, S.M.; Isola, A.M.; Toledo, D.; Rezende, E.; Maia, M.; Magnan, G.B. Enteral nutrition with eicosapentaenoic acid, gamma-linolenic acid and antioxidants in the early treatment of sepsis: Results from a multicenter, prospective, randomized, double-blinded, controlled study: The INTERSEPT study. *Crit. Care* **2011**, *15*. [CrossRef] [PubMed]

24. Schott, C.K.; Huang, D.T. omega-3 fatty acids, gamma-linolenic acid, and antioxidants: Immunomodulators or inert dietary supplements? *Crit. Care* **2012**, *16*, 325. [CrossRef] [PubMed]

Nutrients **2015**, *7*, 5572–5585

25. Zhao, W.; Zhou, S.; Yao, W.; Gan, X.; Su, G.; Yuan, D.; Hei, Z. Propofol prevents lung injury after intestinal ischemia-reperfusion by inhibiting the interaction between mast cell activation and oxidative stress. *Life Sci.* **2014**, *108*, 80–87. [CrossRef] [PubMed]

26. Chen, W.; Jiang, H.; Zhou, Z.Y.; Tao, Y.X.; Cai, B.; Liu, J.; Yang, H.; Lu, C.D.; Zeng, J. Is omega-3 fatty acids enriched nutrition support safe for critical ill patients? A systematic review and meta-analysis. *Nutrients* **2014**, *6*, 2148–2164. [CrossRef] [PubMed]

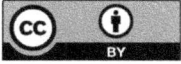

MDPI AG

St. Alban-Anlage 66

4052 Basel, Switzerland

Tel. +41 61 683 77 34

Fax +41 61 302 89 18

http://www.mdpi.com

Nutrients Editorial Office

E-mail: nutrients@mdpi.com

http://www.mdpi.com/journal/nutrients

www.ingramcontent.com/pod-product-compliance
Lightning Source LLC
Chambersburg PA
CBHW051907210326
41597CB00033B/6060